Diabetes is not a piece of cake

Prescribed for family, friends, & co-workers of folks with diabetes.

Revised Third Edition

by Janet Meirelles, R.N.

Certified Diabetes Educator
Certified Health Education Specialist
Member Editorial Board *Diabetes Forecast*

Foreword by: Andrew J. Ahmann, M.D.
Illustrated by: Lee Wright

Lincoln Publishing Incorporated
Lake Oswego, Oregon

Lincoln Publishing Incorporated
http://www.800books4u.com
Tel: (503) 699-1000
Fax: (503) 699-2000
Post Office Box 1499
Lake Oswego, OR 97035-0499
U.S.A.

This book is not intended as a substitute for medical advice of physicians. The reader should regularly consult a physician in matters relating to his or her health and particularly with respect to any symptoms and/or concerns that may require diagnosis or medical attention.

Publisher's Cataloging-in-Publication Data

Meirelles, Janet.
  Diabetes is not a piece of cake :
  prescribed for family, friends, and co-workers of folks
  with diabetes / author, Janet Meirelles ; foreword by,
  Andrew J. Ahmann ; illustrated by, Lee Wright. — Lake
Oswego, OR : Lincoln Pub. Inc., c1994, 1997.

  p. : ill. ; cm.

Includes bibliographical references, glossary, and index.

ISBN: 1-884929-77-X

  1. Diabetes—Popular works.   2. Diabetes.
I. Title.

RC660.4.M   616.462 dc20
                     97-73536

Revised Third Edition
ISBN 1-884929-77-X
Library of Congress Catalogue Number 97-73536

Printed in the United States of America

Foreword

by ANDREW J. AHMANN, M.D.

Diabetes is not a piece of cake... fills a real void in what's available for the family, friends, colleagues, and classmates of people with diabetes. In it you will find out what to do and what to avoid doing to help the person you care about who has diabetes. Subjects discussed vary from social situations to emergencies. From appropriate recipes and going to restaurants, to the symptoms of low and high blood sugar levels, and what you can do.

There are easy to understand and thoughtful explanations of the disease, which will give you an insight into what's happening—you won't merely get dry meaningless instructions.

Even if you have diabetes, and haven't kept up with the latest research, or if you've been too embarrassed to ask questions, there's important information in this book for you too.

There's a thorough glossary, a good index, a supplemental reading list and a summary of resources (like cruises for people with diabetes).

The author also corresponded with, received and reviewed hundreds of questionnaires from people who have diabetes and their family members and shares the insights she gained.

Since your chances of getting diabetes increase with aging, you'll find practical hints on what can be done to reduce those chances— AND, you'll discover reasons that may motivate you to take action now!

This well researched book is pleasant to read, thorough, thoughtful and includes the most recent developments. I hope you will find the time to read it.

DR. AHMANN, in addition to his private practice as an endocrinology specialist, is an Assistant Professor of Medicine and Director of Diabetes Services at Oregon Health Sciences University, School of Medicine. Dr. Ahmann was President of the American Diabetes Association, Oregon Affiliate (1993-94). Dr. Ahmann has received many academic honors, awards, fellowships, and scholarships.

Acknowledgments

My heartfelt thanks to my husband Tom who encouraged me to write this book and helped in a hundred ways to see it through to its completion.

Special thanks to Andrew Ahmann, M.D. (please see bottom of page iii) for his encouragement and Foreword, to James Hansen, M.D., pediatric diabetes specialist and Medical Director of Emanuel Children's Diabetes Center, for his update of children's treatment guidelines, and to Donald Adams, D.D.S., President of the American Academy of Periodontists and Professor and Chairman of Periodontology at OHSU. And, I'm grateful to Lee Wright for his illustrations that humorously show some of the attitudes and pitfalls of having diabetes.

Many thanks also to my colleagues of the Oregon Diabetes Educators who made valuable suggestions. In particular, I wish to thank Nancy Autio, Jody Babson, Sandra Birchall-Jones, Diana Hayes, Martha Hirsch, Patricia Maddix, Carol Schrader, and Marge Thompson.

And thanks also to the hundreds of pen pals from Arabia to Washington who answered my questions, educated me, and told me how much they wanted to share their challenge.

About the Author

Janet Meirelles is a Registered Nurse, a Certified Diabetes Educator and Certified Health Education Specialist. In recent years she has specialized in matters related to diabetes care. She has surveyed hundreds of people who have diabetes and discussed with them their important issues. These issues and experiences led her to write this book about what non-diabetics ought to know and how they can help.

For several years Ms. Meirelles was in charge of a California and Los Angeles County sponsored supplemental services program, an important goal of which was the education about and self-management of diabetes by those within the program. The program she ran received honors and recognition.

Ms. Meirelles is on the Editorial Board of the American Diabetes Association magazine, *Diabetes Forecast* (1997-2000), and has been published therein.

Ms. Meirelles is now in private practice as a diabetes educator and diabetes support group facilitator in the Portland, Oregon area. She is a noted speaker on diabetes and related issues.

Ms. Meirelles is licensed to practice in Oregon, Washington, and California. She graduated from UCLA with a Bachelor of Science in Nursing and from the University of New Mexico with a Bachelor of Arts in Anthropology. Both degrees were awarded with academic honors.

Contents

Chapter 1

Not Everyone With Diabetes Is the Same

Why do some people with diabetes:

> take injections?
> take pills instead of injections?
>
> eat candy?
> don't eat candy?
>
> eat on schedule?
> don't care about a schedule?
>
> test their blood sugar?
> don't test their blood sugar?
>
> become blind or suffer some other complication?
> don't get any complications?

The answers are in this book. We'll discuss what you can do to help your co-worker, friend, or family member with diabetes.

First, I'd like to introduce you to two people I know with diabetes. They're very different but they also have some things in common.

Pat's Story

Pat is a fifty-five year old school teacher who was diagnosed with diabetes five years ago. She was substantially overweight and her blood sugar was four times normal last year, despite taking pills to lower her blood sugar. Her doctor said she was going to have to start insulin if her blood sugar didn't come down. That shocked her into getting her diabetes under control. She started riding her exercise bike and tried to stay on a 1200-calorie diet.

What made following the diet especially hard was that her husband likes pastries and sweets and having those fattening, sugary foods in the house was a constant temptation.

Pat's husband didn't understand why she was making such a big deal about needing to lose weight. He thought she looked fine and she didn't seem sick.

Finally, in late January, Pat got tired of her husband's lack of support for her diabetes program. She found a community evening class on diabetes and brought him along. A good portion of the class dealt with nutrition, especially the importance of avoiding foods high in fat and sugar. He said the class was interesting.

The next morning he offered her jelly donuts—and was surprised at her refusal!

Despite the slow start, Pat's husband did help. The first change was to tell her he didn't need to have pastries and cookies in the house if that made it harder for her to stay on her diet. The second change was to agree to walk with Pat almost every day.

The changes have brought results. Pat lost thirty pounds in eight months and she credits a good deal of that success to her husband's support and cooperation.

John's Story

John is a thirty-nine year old draftsman who also has diabetes. He's had it for thirty years and was only nine when he got it. He injects insulin three times a day, eats meals at scheduled times, avoids sugary foods, exercises every day, and carries candy or other snacks in case his blood sugar gets too low. He also tests his blood sugar five to seven times a day and carries the equipment he needs to do that, plus extra insulin.

John is divorced and lives alone. He often feels that his co-workers and the people he knows socially don't care about his diabetes. At office parties his colleagues only bring food he can't eat and nobody pays attention when he tells them that he needs to eat at a certain time.

He doesn't have any of the serious complications that some people with diabetes get after thirty years but he worries about what still might happen. He hasn't escaped completely unscathed, though. He feels tired and sick when his blood sugar is out of control and often feels sick and tired of being different and having to pay attention to his diabetes. Because he lives alone he feels he doesn't have anyone to support his efforts. Diabetes is expensive too—John spends $100-150 a month just for his supplies.

Pat and John Have Different Kinds of Diabetes

Pat and John got diabetes at different ages. Pat was fifty, John was nine. They also have some very different ways they take care of their diabetes. Pat takes pills, while John takes insulin. Pat still needs to lose some weight, John doesn't.

Type II or Non-Insulin-Dependent Diabetes

Pat has Type II diabetes which used to be called adult onset diabetes and is now called non-insulin-dependent diabetes. She doesn't need insulin because she is still making some of her own. About 95 percent of the people with diabetes have the kind Pat has. They got it as older adults.

Type I or Insulin-Dependent Diabetes

John has Type I diabetes which used to be called juvenile onset diabetes but is now called insulin-dependent diabetes. Fewer than 5 percent of the people with diabetes have Type I.

What Pat and John *do* have in common is that they both need to take steps to keep their blood sugar at normal levels. Also, they could both get the same serious diabetes complications. Lastly, they share a chronic disease that, unless some wonderful cure comes along, will require management for the rest of their lives.

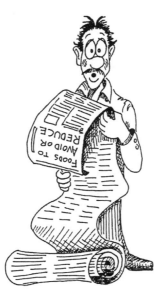

Common Misunderstandings

To help the Pat or John in your life, you may need to unlearn some things about diabetes. Most people think that there are only two things a person with diabetes has to do:

1. Avoid food with sugar.
2. Take insulin shots.

But John eats candy or some form of sugar when his blood sugar gets too low and Pat takes pills instead of insulin shots.

There is a lot more to diabetes than sugar and shots. If you already know more than this, you are better informed about diabetes than 90 percent of the American public. That's according to the people with diabetes who tell me what their friends and family members know or think they know.

Most Diabetes "Teachers" Have Diabetes

The burden of educating people who don't have diabetes has been left almost entirely to the people who have it. Only at social or athletic events do non-diabetics see people with diabetes test or ask for a special food or drink. Then their interest and curiosity are piqued, leading to questions or comments. Some people with diabetes tell me they don't mind telling other people about their disease, while others just want to be left alone to do their diabetes tasks without inquiring minds or offers of help.

Some diabetics[1] tell a friend or family member what they need to know to help keep them safe but that's all they share. They are the exceptions, though. Almost all of the people with diabetes I've spoken to, say it would be a help if others knew more. That's why over three hundred people (from eleven countries) with diabetes answered my questions about what they wished other people knew about living with diabetes. They told me about the things they hate: worrying about complications, pricking a finger for a blood test, taking insulin, and paying for supplies were high on their lists. They had an even longer list of ways their family members, friends, and colleagues make it easier for them to handle their diabetes.

They don't all agree on how they want you to treat them. Some of them want you to treat them like anyone else. Others are pleased and appreciative when you provide special food or ask them how they are doing. It's not hard to learn which of these approaches you should adopt with your loved one, friend, or co-worker. Just ask.

---

[1] Some people consider it politically incorrect to call a person with diabetes a diabetic. However, almost everyone uses "diabetic" in conversation, even those with diabetes. Only two people of the hundreds I asked resented being called a diabetic. Still, in this book, "A person with diabetes" is usually used to avoid giving the idea that the person is just a disease and not a whole person.

This Book Will Get You Started

This book is a guide to those of us who don't have diabetes from those who live with it every waking (and sleeping) hour.

Although someone with diabetes may find parts of this book interesting and the news about recent developments as well as recipes useful, it's not meant to be a comprehensive guide to diabetes management for the person with diabetes or for a person taking total care of a dependent person with diabetes. (See the Suggested Reading List in the Appendix, for detailed diabetes treatment books and magazines).

Since there are different types of diabetes and because your relationship with the person with diabetes may be casual, friendly, or intimate, and because people with diabetes are just as different as you and I, there is often no single right way to handle each situation.

That's why there is some background about diabetes with general medical information in most chapters, followed by suggestions picked up from years of listening to people with diabetes talk about what they wished their friends and family members knew. Included are specific ways in which you can help the person with diabetes, whether by action or by providing emotional support.

Because some readers may want to read the chapters out of order, some basic explanatory material is briefly repeated.

Also, since many of you may be relatives of people with diabetes and may worry that you could get it (actually you could, even if you aren't related to someone with diabetes), there is a chapter called *Do I Have It? Will I Get It?*

I've included my favorite low-sugar and low-fat recipes, but I also urge you to buy or check out recent library books with more selections; these are just a start to get you through a few meals and to be able to bring healthy treats to a social gathering.

The Appendix has summary pages of "how-tos" on recognizing when someone has low blood sugar and what to do about it. You can tear these pages out or photocopy them and place copies in easy-to-see places. That is, if the person you know with diabetes tells you low blood sugar could happen to him or her and doesn't mind posted "reminders."

There are also suggested readings, sources of information, and fun activities in the Appendix, along with a thorough glossary (so you won't need to write down definitions as you go along).

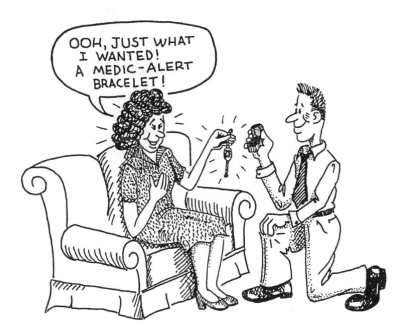

People with diabetes can learn to live well with their disease. John has, despite not having anyone to help with his diabetes anymore. He's learned to do it all himself. And that's hard. He'd love to have someone give some thought to his need to eat on time and avoid sweets. He'd probably love to have you for a friend or office mate after you've read this book.

That's because with your understanding, cooperation, and support you can make an important and positive difference in the care people with diabetes take of themselves. Pat's husband has made that difference.

Chapter 2

The History of Diabetes

The Years Before Insulin

A scribe in Egypt 3,500 years ago described the disease that we know today as diabetes.

The Greeks later called this condition *diabetes mellitus* meaning "honey siphon": "siphon" because of the sufferer's unending urination and "honey" because the urine was sweet-tasting. (You don't want to know how they knew it was sweet but doctors nowadays must be grateful to have labs to send urine specimens to).

In those days, young people who got diabetes wasted away to skin and bones despite ravenous appetites and voracious eating. They urinated a lot because they drank huge amounts of water, but they were still thirsty and wanted more. They got infections that wouldn't clear up, and they became progressively weaker. The only treatment that kept young people alive for a year or two, and older patients alive for longer periods, was a starvation diet. The recommended diet had 500 calories, almost all of that fat and protein, with almost no starches or sugars. Physicians didn't know why that worked, but the less starch and sugar their patients ate, the less sugar they lost in their urine and the slower their weight plunged.

For centuries doctors thought diabetes was a kidney disease. They were wrong about that and really had no clue as to the cause of diabetes until 1890, when Joseph von Mehring and Oskar Minkowsky showed that in animals, removal of the pancreas caused diabetes. They believed that the pancreas produced a substance that controlled the metabolism of food, especially sugars and starches (carbohydrates).

Two decades earlier, Paul Langerhans had described groups of cells in the pancreas, subsequently named the islets of Langerhans, but no one appreciated their importance at the time.

A Baltimore pathologist, E. L. Opie, noticed that in the pancreas of a young woman who had died of diabetes, the islets described by Langerhans were shriveled up.

Given what was known, it seemed logical that if you ground up a pancreas, made a solution, and gave it to experimental animals with diabetes, they might be cured. They tried that but the animals still died of diabetes.

The problem was that the pancreas doesn't produce just the special something that prevents diabetes. It also manufactures digestive enzymes (powerful chemicals that *go through a duct into the intestines* to help digest food). In the pancreas, the clumps of cells that produce enzymes and the ones that produce the "diabetes substance" are separate.

What those early diabetes researchers didn't know is that the magical substance *they were looking for goes directly into the blood*. In our bodies, it never comes in contact with the digestive enzymes the pancreas also makes, so it has no need for protection against those caustic chemicals. By grinding up the whole pancreas, early researchers exposed the vulnerable substance they were looking for to digestive enzymes which destroyed it.

The Discovery of Insulin

In 1921 a young Canadian orthopedic surgeon and medical school instructor with time on his hands read all the available information about diabetes. He was trying to make sense for his medical students of the many conflicting ideas about diabetes. He also had a personal interest—his childhood sweetheart had died of diabetes when the young physician was fifteen years old.

That tragedy is why the twenty-nine year old Canadian, who had begun his university studies in theology to please his parents, switched to medicine in his sophomore year. He graduated as a physician in 1916 and was immediately sent to a field hospital in France. He became a fine surgeon there, was wounded, and showed great compassion for his patients by continuing to operate despite his injury. He came close to bleeding to death and later almost lost an arm to gangrene. After the war, he returned to Canada to start his private practice. To earn enough to survive, he taught physiology to medical students at the University of Western Ontario.

His name was Frederick Banting and he was to get the Nobel Prize for the discovery that changed the treatment of diabetes and brought hope to thousands of its sufferers—the discovery of insulin. While preparing a class on the pancreas, Banting reviewed von Mehring's and Minkowski's work and that of all the other scientists who had contributed what little was known about diabetes. He developed some ideas about how the elusive substance in the pancreas might be found, separated, and used in treatment.

His own colleagues at the University of Western Ontario were not interested in expending resources for such a risky project, but they encouraged Banting to see Dr. J.J.R. MacLeod, a renowned expert in diabetes, at the University of Toronto.

Banting made the long, cold trip to Toronto to beg Dr. MacLeod to help with his idea for separating the substances of the pancreas, but MacLeod turned him down. MacLeod thought it ridiculous that a young doctor with no research experience should tread where great men had failed. Banting persevered, however, and finally MacLeod, who was going away on vacation in the summer of 1921, reluctantly allowed Banting the use of a lab, ten laboratory dogs, and the unpaid help of a research assistant for the two months he would be away.

The research assistant, Charles Best, who had just graduated with a bachelor's degree in biochemistry, was as interested as Banting in finding a cure for diabetes, for he had lost a beloved aunt to the disease. Banting and his ally Best, pooled their savings of less than $500 and on May 17, 1921, they went to work.

They scrimped on food, used up their money for more dogs and supplies, suffered in the hot lab, and made history. These special men— Banting, skilled in surgical techniques, and Best, learned in chemical processes—in only two months with every disadvantage imaginable, produced what they were looking for.

Banting tied off the tiny pancreas ducts through which digestive enzymes go to the intestines. The enzymes backed up, causing the enzyme cells to shrivel and die. Six weeks later, when Banting removed the pancreas, only insulin-producing islets were functioning.

On July 27, 1921, Banting and Best injected the substance they had isolated from the islets into a comatose dog that was dying of diabetes. In hours, the dog was up, energetic, and with no sugar in its urine, but the next day it again lapsed into a diabetic coma and died. Banting and Best then knew that they needed a continuous supply of this miraculous substance, but they also knew that they weren't going to get enough of it from a few dogs. They would need the limitless supply of pancreases they could get from livestock.

To get money to keep their experiments going, Banting sold his car, so his and Best's dozens of trips to stockyards to buy ox pancreases had to be made by streetcar. Keeping the pancreases cool and unspoiled on the slow, hot trips was difficult but Banting and Best got the organs back to the lab safely and were able to extract the precious insulin.

After trying insulin on each other with no ill effects, Banting and Best felt ready to start helping the dozens of dying victims of diabetes in Toronto's hospitals. "Not so fast," said Professor MacLeod, just back from his vacation. He was not amused. Not amused that the two young nobodies should have succeeded where renowned scientists had tried and failed for decades. He was not amused that they hadn't learned a lesson in humility. MacLeod, a recognized expert in diabetes, made them prove everything all over again to his satisfaction.

Happily, everything went well, and MacLeod, instead of further blocking Banting and Best's work, took up the banner to get insulin improved and recognized. He appointed a chemist, James Collip, to help further purify the substance, he changed the name from *isletin* (named after the islets of Langerhans) to the more easily pronounced insulin, and finally, in January 1922, he approved the first testing of insulin on a human.

A mere six months after the lab dog had been briefly revived, a young boy dying of diabetes in a Toronto hospital was offered the chance to be the first person to be treated with insulin. He was bedridden and near death when he and his parents accepted Banting's offer. Within a day, the boy was miraculously better. He was given an injection of insulin every day and was quickly joined by other patients Banting treated.

Meanwhile, Professor MacLeod traveled around Canada and the United States telling physicians and scientists about his team's miraculous discovery of insulin. He gave Banting and Best little credit, though he acknowledged Collip's work in purifying insulin.

In 1923, Banting and MacLeod were awarded the Nobel Prize for medical research. Banting was furious that MacLeod was acknowledged and Best was not. He threatened to refuse the prize but eventually accepted, and gave half of his prize money to Best.

Insulin did not cure diabetes, but it lengthened lives and improved the quality of those lives. The young boy who was first treated with insulin died thirteen years later of pneumonia and complications of diabetes. He would have died in a matter of days or weeks if Banting had not had insulin to give him.

The University of Toronto received a patent for insulin. Although the university never charged drug companies for the use of the process to extract insulin, it did charge a fee to test the purity and activity of the insulin the companies marketed. Profit from the fees went to fund further research by Banting, Best, and Collip.

By the end of 1923, just a little over two years after Banting and Best's first success with the dog, insulin was available in medical centers all over the world. What had once been a rapidly fatal disease to children and young adults had an effective treatment.

Insulin still doesn't cure diabetes, however. It, and the oral medicines since developed for Type II diabetes, only help control the disease. Diabetes needs careful managing for its sufferers to reap the maximum benefit from Frederick Banting and Charles Best's marvelous work.

Other Treatment Discoveries

Wonderful as insulin was, it couldn't do everything. Doctors and patients still needed to find the right combination of insulin and food intake. To do that, they needed to know the blood sugar level as accurately as possible. Remember the physicians in ancient times who used to taste urine as a test for sugar?

Testing for Sugar

Urine Tests

Tasting was eventually followed by the Benedict test—considered the state of the art in its time. It required placing some urine in a test-tube, adding Benedict solution (a blue fluid), and warming the test-tube in a pan of boiling water. After five minutes, the color of the mixture showed whether sugar was in the urine. More than soup got cooked in the kitchens of people with diabetes!

Urine testing continued to get easier. First the cooking became unnecessary—it was replaced by merely dropping a tablet into a urine sample. Finally, the urine test strip for sugar became available. All this test needed was to hold a chemically-treated strip in a stream of urine, shake off the excess, and match the color on the strip to the color chart on the package of strips. This test was easy but it still wasn't very accurate.

For decades, people with diabetes and their physicians based diabetes treatment on home urine sugar tests and occasional laboratory urine and blood tests. But urine tests for sugar give information that can be hours old (while the urine is stored in the bladder) and only indicate high levels, since urine tests can't detect lows.

Blood

Home blood glucose (sugar) testing was a wonderful advance in diabetes treatment. Blood tests identified low, normal, and high blood sugar and gave an immediate result, not one that was hours old. To perform this test, the person pricked a finger, placed a drop of blood on a chemically treated strip, waited one minute, wiped off the strip, waited another minute, and then held the strip up to a color chart on the package just as was done with the urine test strips. With the blood test strip, the person testing knew within 60 mg/dl[1] what his or her blood sugar was two minutes ago!

---

[1] Mg/dl = milligrams per deciliter and reflects the concentration of sugar dissolved in the blood. The normal value varies between 80-120 mg/dl.

The next improvement was the blood sugar meter which can give a specific level of blood sugar like 127, for example, instead of a range of from 120-180.

Improvements in Insulin

Insulin, too, changed from what Banting and Best collected from animal pancreases. Beef and pork insulins frequently caused allergic reactions at the injection site that could lessen their effectiveness. Most insulin used in the United States today is synthetic human insulin made in laboratories.

Back in 1922, there was only one strength of insulin, similar to the regular insulin used today. Its action wore off quickly so several daily injections were necessary. Fifteen years after regular insulin became available, a Danish research team headed by Hagedorn found a combination of insulin with a substance called protamine that slowed insulin's absorption from the tissues. Eventually, mixtures with zinc were developed that were so slowly absorbed that many people got by with only one injection a day.

The newest research has shown that one injection a day, even of long-acting insulin, does not come close to keeping blood sugar in the normal range, as a well-functioning pancreas does. People who want the nearly-normal blood sugar that helps prevent complications are returning to taking three and four injections a day. These more frequent injections combined with the advances in blood sugar testing, have made diabetes control very different from that possible in 1922 when Frederick Banting injected his new insulin into his first patient.

Though Frederick Banting and Charles Best's work has been improved upon, they are truly the heroes in the history of diabetes treatment.

Chapter 3

What Does Diabetes Do?

John's Story—October, 1963

John had been feeling thirsty all the time. He drank tons of juice, soda, and water, but the thirst didn't go away. His mother noticed he was eating a lot more too. "I can't believe how much food a nine-year old boy can put away," she remarked to his father. "He sure doesn't get fat in fact, he looks to me as if he's lost some weight."

John's father said, "He's a growing boy. What do you expect?"

John's father was wrong. It wasn't because he was a growing boy that John was eating and drinking a lot and losing weight.

In the weeks that followed, John drank more fluids than ever and went to the bathroom a lot. He felt tired all the time too, no matter how much sleep he got or how much he ate. He lost thirteen pounds in four weeks.

When his mother realized how much weight he'd lost, she made an appointment with his pediatrician. After hearing the symptoms, John's doctor asked him to go to the bathroom and fill a cup with urine.

A nurse dipped a specially treated paper strip into the sample, and, sure enough, it tested very positive for sugar. The doctor wasted no time. He told John's mother that he was almost sure John had diabetes and that he needed to go to the hospital to get started on insulin.

John spent two weeks in the hospital, getting his dosage of insulin calculated. He also learned about giving himself shots, what an insulin reaction felt like, what to eat, what not to eat, and all kinds of other information about diabetes. He even learned how to do the urine test the nurse had done in the doctor's office. Nowadays he would have been taught how to test his blood, but that wasn't available to patients in 1963.

His mother stayed with him and anxiously tried to take it all in too. In the 1990's, nobody spends two weeks in the hospital if all they need is to adjust their insulin dosage and learn about diabetes.

One reason this long hospital stay was necessary was that in 1963 there was no way people with diabetes could test their own blood at home and have a good idea what their blood sugar was at that moment. They couldn't give accurate, current information to the doctor over the phone and have the doctor easily calculate a safe, effective insulin dosage. Thirty years ago, doctors waited for a laboratory's results of a blood test before deciding how to adjust the amounts of insulin and food for a person newly diagnosed with diabetes. Physicians knew that once the patient went home, they would lose the information from blood tests and have to rely on urine tests until the next office visit when blood could be sent to a lab. Of course, life in the hospital and life outside at home and at school were two different things, so the dosage in the hospital might not be ideal, but that was the best that could be done at that time.

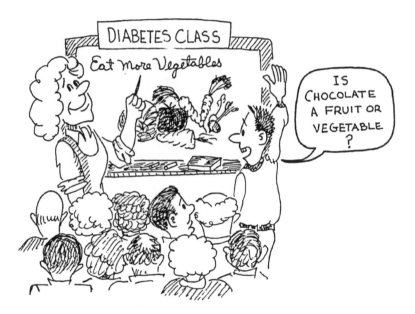

John hated the shots and hated the urine testing. He thought it was very unfair that he couldn't eat candy anymore like other kids. His mom wasn't too happy either. She was given lots of pamphlets and advice about shopping, measuring food, menu planning, how to help John if his blood sugar got low, how to boil the glass syringes, and on and on.

His father wasn't as involved. He did wonder, though, why it had happened to John. No one in *his* family had diabetes. And his wife said nobody on her side had had it either. Wasn't diabetes a hereditary disease?

John and his family learned a lot about diabetes and how to control it, but why John got it is something no one was able to tell them. Even today, scientists have theories but no sure answers about what causes diabetes.

Here are the questions John and his folks asked and the answers they got from the doctor and nurses:

What is diabetes?
Diabetes is a malfunction of the body's use of food that results in a person's being unable to regulate the level of sugar in the blood. Diabetes affects the metabolism of carbohydrates (sugars and starches), protein, and fat but because the primary problem in diabetes is the level of blood sugar and 90 percent of carbohydrates are converted to sugar, carbohydrates are the main concern. To understand what goes wrong, you need to know how the body uses food, especially carbohydrates.

How is food normally used by the body?
The kind of food your body's cells prefer is sugar. Actually, it's a particular kind of sugar called glucose. Cells need sugar or glucose the way your car needs gasoline.

Most of the food you swallow is changed into glucose in the small intestine and then absorbed into the blood where it's carried to every cell in the body.

But getting glucose this far is only equivalent to filling your car's gas tank. That gas still needs to get into the motor, or in the case of glucose, into every cell.

How does the glucose or sugar get into the cell?
What gets the glucose into the cell is insulin, a hormone produced by the pancreas. Hormones are substances that certain body organs produce and release into the blood and that have a specific effect in cells in other parts of the body.[1] The pancreas not only produces the insulin and releases it into the blood, it senses when and how much is needed.

The insulin "escorts" the glucose from the blood into the cell, where it can be used as the cell's food or be stored for future use.

What happens if there is no insulin?
When there is no insulin available, the glucose stays in the blood, and cells don't get their food. When cells don't get their glucose supply, the person starts experiencing the symptoms of diabetes.

---

[1] For example, the hormone epinephrine (Adrenalin) is produced by the adrenal glands which are located near the backbone. When adrenaline is secreted into the blood, it stimulates sweat glands and the heart, dilates air passages in the lungs, and so forth.

What are the symptoms of John's kind of diabetes?[2]

> Increased hunger
> Weight loss
> Tiredness
> Infections
> Increased thirst
> Increased urination
> Blurred vision

How can a person have increased hunger, eat more, and still lose weight?
When cells do not get the food they need, the body "thinks" it's starving. It tries to get more food by stimulating the sense of hunger. Unfortunately, eating more doesn't help because more food is just changed into more glucose, which makes the blood even more sugary. When that doesn't work, the body tries to get glucose from its protein supplies, most of which are in muscle tissue. The liver then converts that protein into glucose. But, again, the glucose level in the blood just goes higher. As muscles waste away, it's possible to actually lose weight despite eating extra food.

Where does tiredness come in?
Along with the hunger and weight loss comes tiredness. Eight hours' sleep, vitamin pills, pots of coffee: nothing seems to help. Cells without food are cells that don't want to move muscles.

Why do people with diabetes get more infections?
Muscle cells are not the only cells that are going without glucose. The cells in the immune system, especially white blood cells and antibodies, are unable to work, so germs and viruses may cause frequent, slow-healing infections.

These are the consequences of the cells not getting glucose. Meanwhile, with nowhere to go, the glucose accumulates in the blood. A different set of consequences results from the build-up of excess glucose.

Too much glucose in the tissues is an ideal breeding ground for many bacteria and fungi. That's why vaginal and urinary tract infections are common at the time diabetes is diagnosed or any other time when blood sugar stays high for too long.

---

[2] There is another kind of diabetes with less obvious symptoms. That diabetes will be described later in the chapter.

Why does diabetes make a person feel thirsty and urinate more?
Without insulin, the blood glucose level can rise to ten times normal. Since even double the normal range is harmful, the body tries to get rid of the excess glucose. The kidneys try to flush it out by making more urine. Thirst is increased to get more water for the kidneys' increased urine production. The person drinks more and urinates more. This urine has a lot of glucose in it. In fact, this is where much of the glucose that couldn't get into the cells is lost.

The body's attempt to get rid of the sugar by making sweet urine is still not enough to get the blood sugar to normal levels. The kidneys only start making extra urine when the glucose in the blood is about double the normal level, which is too high to maintain a healthy cell environment. To lower it further requires medication, exercise, and diet change.

Why is blurred vision a symptom of diabetes?
What does sugar in the blood have to do with eyesight?
High sugar levels in the blood can also cause blurred vision when increased urination depletes the body of fluids. That gradually causes the lens in the eye to shrink. Later, when the body's water balance normalizes, the lens of the eye swells as fluid slowly re-enters from the blood. It doesn't matter if the lens is getting shriveled or plumping up—both conditions result in blurred vision. This is not a permanent condition. It's just a bad idea to think new eye glasses will clear things up. Weeks may go by before the lens is again normal.

Does everyone with diabetes experience these symptoms?
No. Extreme thirst, hunger, weight loss, and frequent urination are the symptoms of diabetes in a person who is producing little or no insulin. This type of diabetes is called Type I diabetes, or insulin-dependent diabetes.

Who gets Type I or insulin-dependent diabetes?
Type I diabetes occurs most often in children and young adults. Only about ten percent of people with diabetes have Type I. But a person under forty years of age newly diagnosed with diabetes is likely to have this type. John has Type I diabetes.

What other types of diabetes are there?
Type II diabetes, or non-insulin-dependent diabetes, is the most common type of diabetes. It occurs when the pancreas produces some insulin, but perhaps not quite enough, or when the insulin is not being used effectively. It progresses more slowly and may not have the dramatic

symptoms of Type I diabetes. It is more common in people over forty, although children or young adults can also get it.

Some pregnant women get a diabetes called gestational diabetes (which is much like Type II diabetes). It's due to the effect of pregnancy hormones that disturb the usual balance of food and insulin. It's temporary in 97 percent of women who get it, though it usually recurs in any subsequent pregnancies and, not infrequently, can recur later in life as Type II diabetes.

There are also other kinds of diabetes due to disease of the pancreas or its surgical removal, glandular problems, and medications that raise blood sugar, such as cortisone.[3] These conditions either decrease or eliminate the supply of insulin or make it less effective.[4]

Does eating sugar cause diabetes?
No. If a person does not have diabetes, the pancreas can produce enough insulin, and any amount of sugar will be used effectively or stored as fat. Only a pancreas that is already damaged or a body that can't use insulin well has a problem with sugar.

Is diabetes contagious?
No. It is not at all like a cold or the measles.

What causes diabetes?
Diabetes is caused by both heredity and environment. Type I, the kind John has, is believed to be caused by a genetic defect that predisposes an individual to overreact to a viral infection. Perhaps some other stress to the immune system is also involved. When these factors are present, the insulin-producing cells of the pancreas may be destroyed. One million Americans living today have had enough insulin cells destroyed to get Type I diabetes.[5]

Type II diabetes is more likely to strike a person who has other family members with diabetes, especially if that person is carrying around a lot of extra fat. Frequently the pancreas is doing just fine and is pumping out lots of insulin but the cells are not paying attention to the insulin. The cells "resist" the insulin, and excess fat is usually at least partly to blame

---

[3] Cortisone is sometimes the only medication that is effective in treating asthma, lupus, and arthritis.

[4] *Diabetes insipidus* is a very different condition that has nothing to do with the pancreas or insulin use. It involves the pituitary gland and the kidneys. The word *diabetes (siphon)* is shared because both diseases cause increased urination.

[5] It is estimated that there are 13 million people with Type II diabetes, which does not result from an immune system problem.

for that resistance. In fact, eight out of ten people with Type II diabetes are overweight.

Along with heredity, viral infection, and excess body fat, there is a fourth contributing cause to diabetes: stress. Actually, both the virus and the excess fat are stresses to the body, but we usually think of stress as a psychological burden. When we lose a loved one, a job, or our health, we call that stress. If too much is expected of us, we experience stress. Any change in our lives is a stress that requires the body to adapt.

Help in dealing with stress comes in the form of three hormones: epinephrine (Adrenalin), cortisol (similar to cortisone), and insulin. All three make it easier for us to flee or fight some danger in our surroundings. Epinephrine raises the blood pressure and heart rate so our muscles can get extra blood to run or fight. Cortisol helps the body change stored protein and fat into sugar for use by the muscles as fuel. Insulin, of course, gets that sugar into the muscle cells.

If everything works well, the exercise of escaping or fighting uses up the sugar, and when the danger is over, the body returns to its normal state. Some stress is a normal condition, and our bodies are well equipped to handle both good stress (eustress) and bad stress (distress). But too much for too long can overtax the body's coping mechanisms. If stress continues at high levels, the extra blood sugar that the cortisol calls up may be more than some weakened pancreases can handle. If not enough insulin can be made or if insulin resistance is present, high blood sugar becomes constant and diabetes results.

What happens if someone with Type I Diabetes doesn't take insulin?
Because insulin is so essential to the body's survival, a lack of it, or even a seriously low level, causes tiredness, hunger, weight loss, infections, increased thirst, increased urination, and blurred vision quickly. In days, or at most a couple of weeks, people with Type I diabetes start reporting all or almost all of these symptoms. If they do not get diagnosed and get insulin, they eventually lose consciousness and die.

Some people with diabetes take pills instead of insulin, why can't John?
John is not producing insulin. This is evident because when his urine was tested, it contained two things that shouldn't have been there: sugar and ketones. Anybody with diabetes can have sugar in their urine, but ketones, a waste product of burning fat, are almost always a sign that the person has a severe shortage of insulin—so severe that the body is unable to use the sugar in the blood and must burn stored fat to survive.

How is the onset of Type II diabetes different?

Type II diabetes comes on more slowly. Sometimes it is not caused by a lack of insulin. In fact, some people with Type II diabetes produce greater than usual levels of insulin, but they don't use it efficiently. The end result is that the glucose still accumulates in the blood and the cells still don't get the food they need to function well. Thus all of the symptoms of Type I diabetes can also be felt by people with Type II. Usually, however, because of the slow onset of Type II diabetes, people with this type don't feel thirsty or lose weight.

More commonly, a person with Type II diabetes will complain of tiredness. But since this is not unusual in the overweight and those over fifty, it can be overlooked as a symptom of diabetes. People just think, "Of course I'm tired. I'm getting old."

In fact, some people have Type II for years before it's diagnosed. They may actually suffer a long-term complication—such as an infection that doesn't heal, especially a foot infection, or leg pain or numb feet—before they're told they have diabetes. These long-term complications of diabetes usually mean that the person has had high blood sugar levels for at least five years.

The symptoms of Type II diabetes are:

Tingling, numbness, or pain in legs or feet
Slow healing of cuts and sores
Frequent skin infections or itchy skin
Tiredness or drowsiness

What are the complications of diabetes?

The complications most people think about first are blindness, kidney failure, and foot amputations. These are the end results of damage to the retina of the eye, the kidney, and the nerves and blood vessels of the legs.[6]

People are less likely to associate heart attacks and strokes with diabetes, but years of high blood sugar together with high cholesterol levels in the blood can lead to a waxy build-up (plaque) inside blood vessels. A blood vessel in the heart that is significantly narrowed by plaque eventually won't allow enough blood to get through. When the blood carrying essential oxygen and food can't get to the part of the heart that it supplies, that part dies. That's what is called a heart attack. A blocked

---

[6] See Chapter 7 on complications.

blood vessel in the brain can mean a stroke. Strokes and heart attacks are all too frequently complications of diabetes. In one hospital I worked in, there were more patients with diabetes on the heart disease unit than in the diabetes unit.

Part of the problem is that people with diabetes tend to have more cholesterol and other fats in their blood that make up plaque. Even though John is very young, it's not too early for him to control the amount of fats, especially saturated fats, that can increase cholesterol in the blood. To do this he should eat less animal fat.

Nerves in many parts of the body can be damaged and are the basis for complications ranging from mild to life threatening.

Can anyone with diabetes get complications?
Yes. People with Type I diabetes are not the only ones at risk of getting complications. Just because a person is producing some insulin and had a slow onset of diabetes does not mean complications don't occur.

There are some differences between Type I and Type II diabetes, but the danger of high blood sugar is there for both. The longer the person has diabetes with higher-than-normal blood sugar, the greater the chance of getting the complications.

Here is an overview of the similarities and differences in the two types of diabetes:

	Type I	Type II
Number of US cases	1 million	14 million plus
Age when usually diagnosed	Under 40	Over 40
Speed of onset	Days-weeks	Weeks-years
Need to take insulin	Always	Sometimes
Can treat with pills	Never	Often
Diet & exercise part of treatment	Always	Always
Can get complications	Yes	Yes

Is there a cure for diabetes?
The only present cure for diabetes is a pancreas transplant. Such transplants are done in only a few medical centers in the United States. Pancreas transplants require continuous medication to suppress rejection of the new organ. They are still considered experimental by many insurance companies although they have been done for twenty-seven years.

The last ten years have seen enormous progress in the number of transplants done with successful outcomes. Presently the five-year survival rate of transplanted pancreases is fifty to seventy percent.

Some centers are also trying to transplant only the beta cells that make the insulin. Such transplants are called islet cell transplants and are so new they are considered an experimental treatment by everybody.

For most people with diabetes, neither of these options is possible because of the surgical and rejection risks, plus the huge expense.

Surgery is always risky, especially with a patient who has a chronic illness with impaired healing ability, as is the case with diabetes. In addition, the medications that keep the pancreas from being rejected have many unpleasant side effects. They cause fluid retention, make the skin fragile, and inhibit the body's ability to fight infection. And they must be taken for the rest of the person's life.

The surgery and the medications required afterward are, at best, only partially reimbursed by insurance. Frequently, companies refuse to pay any part of the expense on the grounds that pancreas transplants are experimental.

But the work being done despite these road blocks indicates that progress is being made and we can reasonably hope for a cure in the foreseeable future.

Does diabetes ever go away by itself?
No, but there may be a temporary remission. In about 20 percent of recently diagnosed people with Type I (insulin-dependent) diabetes, the need for injected insulin may decrease or even stop for a short while. Usually this "honeymoon phase" lasts a few weeks, although there have been a few cases in which it continued for two or more years before the insulin dosage had to be increased or restarted.

One theory about why this occurs is that in some people at the time of diagnosis, the insulin-producing beta cells that are not yet dead are too exhausted to carry the full load formerly borne by millions of healthy cells. These "exhausted" cells no longer produce insulin. After a few weeks of insulin injections, though, during which no demands are being placed on the pancreas's beta cells, they get a second wind and can produce enough or nearly enough insulin without injections—for a while.

Cases of people in the "honeymoon phase" are probably responsible for reports of miraculous "cures" and successes with alternate therapies. The news of someone going off insulin is a much bigger story than the person's eventual relapse, so you probably would never hear that insulin later was needed again—permanently.

Chapter 4

Treatments: Different Pokes for Different Folks

John has Type I diabetes and takes insulin three times a day. But even though everyone with Type I diabetes needs insulin, not everyone takes three injections a day.

Pat, whom you also met in Chapter 1, has Type II diabetes. There is even more variation in the treatment of her kind of diabetes. Some people with Type II diabetes, like Pat, take a pill to help reduce their blood sugar. Others need insulin, and still others control their disease with diet and exercise alone.

What makes the difference? What else do people do to control their disease?

Here are questions that Pat, John, or John's parents asked at one time or another about treating diabetes.

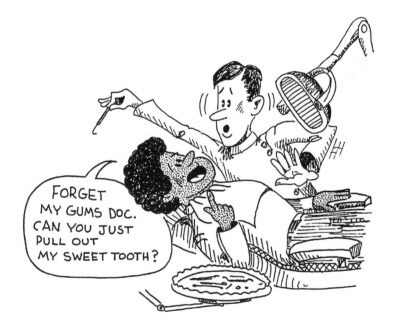

What is the treatment for Type I diabetes?

People with little or no insulin production need to inject insulin at least once a day. At present, there is no other way to get insulin reliably into the body. When insulin was a new medicine, there was only one kind, which we now call regular insulin. Its effects lasted only a few hours, so several injections were necessary every day. Fortunately, insulin is now also formulated into long-lasting and intermediate-acting types that can keep the blood glucose stable for many hours, so not everyone has to take three or four injections a day.

Most people with Type I diabetes take two injections a day, one before breakfast and another before dinner. But some people take three or four, or more.

Why do some people take more than two injections a day?

For some people, two injections a day are not enough. Their blood sugar cannot be kept in the normal range with a two-shot schedule. They may get a very high blood sugar at certain times when the last dose has worn off.

People who have very changeable blood sugar or who want to keep it in as near a normal range as possible take three or four or more injections a day. Some people vary the dosage, depending on how high or low their blood glucose level is. For them, there is no standard dosage of insulin that will consistently keep their blood sugar in a nearly normal range.

Other factors that have to do with preferences and the doctor's judgment also affect the insulin schedule. (More about this later).

How is the treatment for Type II diabetes different?

People with Type II diabetes produce their own insulin. It may not be quite enough or it may not be used efficiently, but they are not experiencing a complete absence of insulin. However, they may have one or more of four other problems.

1. One problem has to do with an incorrect signal being given to the liver. In people without diabetes, when insulin levels are high (after meals, for example), the liver removes glucose from the blood, and stores it in a form called glycogen. When the insulin level is low, as it typically is between meals, another hormone produced by the pancreas, called glucagon, signals the liver to break down the stored glycogen, turns it back into glucose, and releases it back into the bloodstream.

In Type II diabetes, the pancreas continues to release glucagon which then signals the liver to release glucose when levels are already too high. Adding that glucose to the glucose from the food means that the blood sugar goes up even higher. One's own insulin should regulate this process, but it fails to do so.

Metformin (Glucophage) acts on the liver to reduce the release of glucose.
2. If the pancreas can no longer produce enough insulin to get glucose into cells, the solution may be drugs called sulfonyulureas. These are "pancreas stimulators." Common ones are Glucotrol, Glynase, Micronase, and Amaryl. If these don't work insulin is the next step.
3. The third problem with Type II diabetes may be that insulin is not released quickly enough after eating. Usually, getting the new batch of glucose from the meal out of the blood and into the cells should take no more than three hours. If the insulin release is delayed, the blood sugar stays high longer than it should. The medication for this problem is Acarbose (Precose), which slows down the digestion of some carbohydrates so a slow pancreas has a chance to keep up.
4. The fourth problem is resistance to insulin. It occurs in the cell, especially muscle cells, which should remove glucose from the blood and restock muscles for the next time energy is called for. A person could produce plenty of insulin and still have high blood sugar (and feel lack of energy) if this were the problem. In 1997, troglitazone (Rezulin) became the first medication approved in the U.S. to reduce insulin resistance in the muscles.

Are pills always necessary for Type II diabetes?
Changes in lifestyle can lessen insulin resistance and help the body's natural insulin work more efficiently. (1) One of these is to lose weight. (2) Another is to reduce the quantity of food and (3) the amount of carbohydrate in that food. That means smaller, more frequent meals with little or no sweets or otherwise reducing carbohydrates (see Chapters 10 & 11). (4) Exercise is the fourth beneficial change.

If diet, weight loss, and exercise sufficiently reduce the need for more insulin at meals or reduce insulin resistance and the natural insulin keeps blood sugar in the normal range, no pills or shots are needed.

If, for whatever reason, the blood glucose won't come down or starts creeping back up while taking pills, insulin injections are the next step. For people with Type II diabetes, one injection a day may be enough to help the pancreas so that it can manage to keep the blood sugar under control the rest of the time.

How does the doctor know if a person needs pills or insulin and how much?
The decision of what medicine is best, is based on the patient's blood sugar level. Blood sugar tests used to be done only occasionally. The doctor would draw the patient's blood from a vein during an office visit and send it to a laboratory. A day or so later, the patient and the doctor

knew what the blood glucose was at the time it was drawn. Imagine having to take your car to your mechanic every time you wanted to know if it needed gas and having to wait a day or two to find out how much?

Nowadays, patients can test their own blood sugar levels several times a day instead of only a few times a year. That means they can test at home, keep track of the results, and phone their physician with the levels, allowing the doctor to change the dosage more frequently and to base the change on more than a single office visit and lab test. Knowing *when* the blood sugar is high or low is as important as knowing the level. Diabetes management has improved enormously since patients have been able to test their own blood wherever they are and get the results immediately.

Whether the person with diabetes is three or eighty-three, has Type I or Type II, uses insulin or takes pills, the ability to test blood glucose and make adjustments means that he or she can maintain a much more normal blood glucose. Even if the person takes neither pills nor insulin, a rising blood sugar can be an early signal that there is an infection or some other body stress occurring, or it can simply mean that pills or insulin are now needed. In either case, the physician can be called and whatever is necessary can be done—early.

Why can't you test urine instead of blood for sugar?
For decades, urine tests were the only do-it-yourself tests available to detect higher than normal blood sugar. But people with diabetes need to know more than that their blood sugar is high. Low and normal blood sugar are useful to know about too, but urine tests for sugar can't give this information. Kidneys only remove *excess* sugar; there is no change in urine when blood sugar is low.

Normally, there is no sugar in urine. Kidneys start removing excess glucose from the blood only after blood glucose reaches twice the normal level. So no sugar in the urine can mean that the blood sugar is anywhere from 0 to around 200[1] which includes low, normal, and moderately high blood sugar. A urine sugar test is not very helpful.

A test that tells when blood sugar is low or is heading there is very important.

Why is it important to know when blood sugar is getting low?
Even though a lower-than-normal blood sugar may sound good because it's high blood sugar that causes long term complications, it is neither healthy nor comfortable to have low blood sugar. Low blood sugar means

---

[1] The level of blood sugar at which kidneys allow sugar to escape in urine varies. The average is 180 to 200. That average gets higher with age so the older we are the less useful a urine sugar test is.

the cells aren't getting enough glucose, which brings on unpleasant symptoms such as sweatiness, shakiness, and hunger, that signal the sugar shortage.

A low blood sugar *can even be life threatening if the brain becomes so deprived of glucose that the person becomes unconscious and has an accident. Continued brain cell deprivation can even cause a fatal coma.* Very low blood sugar is so serious that the pancreas produces a hormone called glucagon to try to correct the problem. Glucagon tells the liver to release stored glucose when the supply in the blood is low. People with diabetes don't usually rely on this emergency back-up, though; they eat or drink something fast—at the first sign of sweatiness, shakiness, or hunger. (See Chapter 8 on low blood sugar and how to help when it happens).

When people had only urine tests to check for sugar, they never knew if they were already low or were getting into the low range. It was frequently an unpleasant surprise and, as mentioned above, could be dangerous. So it was a real boon when a test came along that showed accurate highs *and* lows and that when repeated after a short time, could give an idea of what direction the blood sugar was moving.

The urine test for sugar is definitely a thing of the past. However, there is a urine test for ketones that is a very useful tool.

What are ketones and why do you test for them?
Ketones are the by-products of the body using stored fat. They are produced when the body desperately needs a source of energy because sugar is not getting into the cells. The usual reason the cells are not getting enough sugar is because there isn't enough insulin to "escort" it inside.[2]

When there is a shortage of insulin, the body starts changing stored fat into sugar in an attempt to provide food of some kind to prevent cell starvation. The problem with using fat as a primary energy source, is that it gives off toxic chemicals called ketones. They are generally harmful, cause nausea and vomiting, and are hard for the body to get rid of.

Luckily, there is an easy urine test that will show whether ketones are being produced so that steps can be taken to stop this cycle. By dipping a special, chemically treated strip into fresh urine and then comparing the color of the strip to a color chart, one can tell if there are any ketones and if there are, whether the amount is small, moderate, or large.

The presence of ketones usually means that the diabetes is out of con-

---

[2] Another cause for the cells not getting enough sugar is that the person may not be eating enough carbohydrate. This is uncommon, however, and only occurs if people are on very restricted diets or during a fast or famine.

trol and calls for some corrective measures. Taking more insulin and drinking a lot of water are usually the first steps. The insulin makes it possible for the body to use the sugar that's available and to stop using fat. The water helps the kidneys flush out the ketones in urine, just as they do with excess sugar. The more help the kidneys get (by drinking lots of water), the faster the body gets rid of the ketones.

What happens if ketones keep accumulating?

When ketones keep accumulating, a condition called ketoacidosis occurs.[3] The more urine the kidneys make to wash out the ketones, the more dehydrated the person becomes, and the higher the ketone concentration in the blood becomes.

If not caught early, ketoacidosis requires hospitalization to replace fluids and get the body back in balance with the correct concentration of insulin and sugar.

Furthermore, the initial shortage of insulin is often due to an illness that requires extra sugar to supply energy to fight the illness. To accommodate that need, the liver puts out stored sugar. That extra sugar is what usually makes the normal amount of insulin insufficient and starts the whole process of the body metabolizing fat and producing ketones as a by-product. The illness that started the whole process needs to be diagnosed and treated.

Usually the illness is an infection of some sort but it can also be a heart attack or any other condition that places a stress on the body. Even emotional stress can trigger the liver to release sugar. Whatever the trigger, it must be found and dealt with.

If testing blood sugar is so useful, doctors must tell everybody with diabetes to test often and call them often with the results, right?

Not really. Not everybody needs to test several times a day. For example, for the person with Type II diabetes who is maintaining normal blood sugar with diet and exercise, once a day at different times each day, or possibly once every other day at varied times may be enough. It's generally accepted practice to tell people who take insulin to test before every injection to be sure their blood sugar level is not already low. This is considered a safety practice.

---

[3] Ketoacidosis is explained further in Chapter 9 on high blood sugar.

It's Hard to Compare

There are as many combinations of blood testing frequency and times as there are schedules and ways of taking insulin. This variety makes a diabetes care plan very flexible.

The reason I bring this up is that people with diabetes tell me they are frequently challenged by their friends and family with statements like "George has diabetes and his doctor doesn't tell him to ___." You fill in the blank. But George's doctor may have different goals for George, or George may have a problem only he and his doctor and family know about, or George may not be telling you what his doctor *really* told him to do.

Given the many treatment choices, it is not useful to compare and challenge the doctor's instructions of your friend or family member who has diabetes with anyone else's diabetes management. Here are four doctors and their patients, each with a different treatment plan.

Four Doctors: Four Treatment Plans

Doctor Smith puts most of her newly diagnosed Type II patients on a strict weight reduction diet before she starts them on any diabetes medication. She has them check their blood sugar before breakfast.

Dr. Jones prescribes oral medication for patients newly diagnosed with Type II diabetes and sends them to a dietitian for instruction in a diet with limited portions and no sugar. He wants them to check their blood sugar three times a day, two hours after meals.

Dr. Lewis tells patients newly diagnosed with Type II diabetes to lose weight by reducing fat and sugar and by exercising vigorously six days a week. He has them test their blood before breakfast and before and after exercise for two weeks and report to him by phone.

Dr. Day tells newly diagnosed patients with Type I diabetes to take two insulin injections a day, follow a diabetic exchange diet, and test their blood sugar before every shot and at bedtime.

Which of these doctors is right? It depends.

Treatment Depends on Several Factors

Treatment depends on whether the patient has Type I or Type II diabetes. It depends on the patient's weight. It depends on what the doctor knows about the patient's resources and how those resources will make it easier or harder for the patient to follow certain aspects of a particular diabetes plan. It depends on what the doctor's training was and how rigorous he or she believes diabetes treatment has to be. It depends on the latest scientific data the doctor may have read or heard at a recent seminar.

Nearly everything about diabetes management "depends."

Weight

The patient's weight can have an impact on what medications, activity, and diet the physician prescribes.

As you can see from the four doctors' diet instructions above, there isn't one "right" diet. Some patients need to limit sugar and carbohydrates while others need to reduce fat and calories.

Reducing fat and calories is especially important for people over forty who get diabetes. Eighty percent or so of them are overweight. But if a doctor has been seeing a patient for years, and for years has been suggesting that the patient lose weight without success, the doctor may give up in that area and concentrate on other areas of treatment, like reducing sweets, eating at scheduled times, and taking medication.

Patient Resources

A patient's resources often dictate what a physician can and can't include in a diabetes plan. When we say "resources" we usually think of financial means. But resources also cover the patient's lifestyle (which includes family help, job demands, and nearness to medical facilities), emotional health, and mental and/or physical skills that could make some aspect of the diabetes plan impossible or impractical.

Poor Vision

Some patients are very able to mentally make responsible decisions but have poor eyesight. Actually, the visually impaired and even those who are completely blind are less dependent than you might expect. There are blood sugar testing meters that "talk" and insulin-measuring devices that allow accurate dosing without the aid of a sighted human helper. There are two areas that the visually handicapped can't manage alone, however: checking their feet for white or reddened areas that could indicate a foot infection and (usually) transportation to doctors. Your help with these could be much appreciated.

Patient Resistance

Some patients simply will not stop smoking or drinking to excess. Others won't exercise regularly, lose weight, reduce sugar, or take insulin. Perhaps they've tried to diet or stop smoking or drinking in the past, but they've failed. Maybe they just aren't willing to fail again. For some people, taking insulin shots is so fear-provoking that they can't bring themselves to do it. In the case of a patient with Type I diabetes who needs insulin to survive, the fear of death eventually overcomes the fear of the needle. But in the case of a patient with Type II diabetes whose blood sugar is high on oral medication but who can stay alive without insulin, the threat of future complications may not be enough to make that person give himself or herself injections.

Lecturing and threats of complications are the usual tools health professionals use to overcome patient resistance. Counseling and behavior modification are less often recommended but can produce good results with most resistant patients. Often the problem is finding money for them.

Learning Problems

Rigidity and fear are not the only barriers to a patient taking care of herself or himself. Sometimes the person is not intellectually capable of learning the skills necessary to treat diabetes effectively. Learning deficiencies can prevent a person from using a blood sugar meter, following a diabetic meal plan, or accurately measuring an insulin dose. For this person, a plan may have to be simplified to "Don't eat sugary foods and don't eat a lot of food at one meal." Sometimes a visiting nurse, friend, or relative must fill insulin syringes, give injections, or test blood, at least for a time. If no dependable professional or loved one can help at home, the person may have to live in a group home where a care giver can do the essential diabetes tasks.

Blood Sugar Testing

Testing blood sugar is a key aspect of diabetes treatment that varies tremendously according to the physician's beliefs and the patient's resources. Frequently, all the factors already mentioned influence when, where, how, and if a patient tests. Another factor is whether the patient thinks it's worth the time and money.

Testing Without Knowing Why, Is Not Enough

Blood sugar testing sometimes seems a waste of time to people who prick their fingers, do the test, fill in their logs, and show three months of tests to their doctor during an office visit, only to have the doctor barely glance at the figures. Or sometimes the doctor looks at the numbers and changes the medication dosage without telling the patient what he or she noticed that justified the change. That's a pity.

The more the physician involves the patient in the decision-making process and the better the person understands the balance of insulin, exercise, and food, and how they affect the blood sugar, the more likely he or she is to learn how to control each factor and to appreciate the importance of blood sugar tests.

Many studies have shown that blood sugar testing alone does not improve blood sugar control because the essential factor is not the testing, but the patient's knowing what to do with the results of the tests. If the physician or a diabetes educator can convey the importance of blood testing as a *tool*, it can change the patient's perception of the chore: what once seemed an apparently imperious demand can turn into a meaningful aid in the patient's getting and keeping control of the disease.

When to Test

As part of the diabetes management plan, a physician recommends what times of day the patient should test. Some doctors believe that the most important blood sugar reading is the one before breakfast. That's called the fasting blood sugar because the patient has had nothing to eat (fasted) all night while asleep. A fasting blood sugar level above 126 is now considered the threshold for diagnosis of diabetes. Prior to June 1997, the number was 140, 70 to 110 would be ideal.

Other doctors say that it's pretty easy to get the fasting blood sugar under control, but it's the ones after meals (post-prandial), which stay high for hours, that need to be brought to light and be dealt with. These physicians want their patients to test one to two hours after meals and to have a blood sugar level under 180.[4] If the level is higher, the patients know they ate too much at the previous meal or ate too much carbohydrate, maybe even some concentrated form they may not have known was in the food, such as honey or corn syrup. Those patients are given information about modifying their food intake.

---

[4] Whether it's one or two hours that the doctor says to wait before testing, be consistent about that time and start the timer when you *start* eating.

How Often To Test

Doctors usually order more frequent blood testing if the patient is on diabetes medication, whether that is pills, insulin, or both. That's because medication lowers blood sugar, sometimes too much. By testing, a person can find out if the level is low or is likely to get too low and can eat something to correct or prevent it. Times when that is likely to happen are when the person exercises, skips or delays a meal, or eats less than usual.

How frequently the doctor orders blood testing may depend on other factors. A recent change in medication, diet, or exercise usually requires closer monitoring of blood sugar, at least temporarily.

Another factor in the frequency of blood testing is the patient's previous experience: recent excessively high or low blood sugar levels may indicate that more monitoring is necessary. Some patients have stable blood sugar that varies little once they can control the portion sizes of meals. Others can adhere to a strict diet, exercise the prescribed amount, take the same dosage of medication, and still have high and low blood sugar readings seemingly without rhyme or reason. Frequent testing for these people helps them predict and prevent some of those highs and lows and may help them discover the causes. And if the cause can be discovered and eliminated, the person can test less frequently.

More frequent testing is also desirable when a person has lost some or all sensitivity to the signs of low blood sugar. Normally, low blood sugar makes a person feel sweaty, shaky, hungry, and nervous. These are signs that some food or juice is needed to raise blood sugar. Some people do not have this warning. It could be because they have had low blood sugar too often and have thereby depleted the alarm hormones that give the signal, or they may be taking a medicine that blocks these hormones. The first they may know of a low blood sugar is when a paramedic is leaning over them and they're being given glucose by vein. For them, testing whenever there is a possibility of low blood sugar, such as after exercise, is essential.

Blood Sugar Testing and Lifestyle

A patient's lifestyle can affect how often a physician prescribes blood sugar testing. For example, a person who lives alone may need to test more frequently because there's no one around to help spot symptoms of a low blood sugar and run to get a glass of juice.

Another good candidate for frequent blood sugar testing is someone who operates machinery or has some other job of special responsibility, such as caring for young children. Such people have to be extra careful about preventing muddled thinking, disorientation, or the worst-case scenario-a loss of consciousness—that very low blood sugar can cause.

Blood Sugar Testing and Financial Resources

Another factor in deciding how often blood testing is done is money—especially the lack of it. We hate to admit that people's health can be compromised by the dollar, but it is. Blood testing strips are about 65 cents each. A patient who is not taking insulin frequently has no insurance reimbursement for blood testing supplies. Or the person may not have insurance. Even if the patient's medical condition dictates testing four times a day, if the $80.60 a month isn't there, the patient can't test.[5]

Past Experience of a Physician Influences Treatment

In addition to the strengths and limitations that the patient brings to the treatment options, the physician also has experiences that have an impact on diabetes management decisions. The training of the doctor has a lot to do with the diabetes treatment he recommends.

For many years a debate raged in the medical community regarding the usefulness of insisting that the patient try to maintain a normal blood sugar level. Many physicians, backed by the American Diabetes Association, believed that high blood sugar was responsible for the complications that people got after decades with diabetes. These doctors prescribed diabetes programs designed to keep blood sugar as close to normal as possible. These regimens were a lot of work for the doctor and the patient. They required discipline and cost more. The proponents claimed that the effort paid off. But not all doctors agreed.

The dissenting physicians felt that very high blood sugar and ketoacidosis should be prevented, but that more than this was not very beneficial. They believed that complications would develop regardless of how aggressive the treatment plan was, so why burden the patient with extra work and expense?

Both groups of physicians relied on their training and experience to back up their conclusions. Until recently there wasn't a clinical study that unequivocally proved either point of view. Now there is.

---

[5] For more on this subject, see Chapter 6 on insurance and costs.

What We Know Now

In June 1993 at the American Diabetes Association's annual convention, the results of the *Diabetes Control and Complications Trial (DCCT)* were presented for the first time. The statistics from this nine-year study showed that the incidence and severity of complications can be significantly reduced by keeping the blood sugar level as close to normal as possible. The data that back up this conclusion include photographs of the interior of eyes and chemical tests that show kidney function. These are both objective measurements of physical status, not merely opinions.

Proof of the blood sugar level was provided by objective laboratory tests, not by patients monitoring on portable meters and recording the results. The blood sugar level was determined from a blood sample drawn in the doctor's office or clinic and sent to a laboratory. The laboratories performed a relatively new test that reflects how often blood sugar has been high over the last three months.[6] The test measures the amount of glucose that has "stuck" to the hemoglobin part of red blood cells during the lifetime of the cells, and cannot be altered by anything the patient does a day or two before the blood is drawn.[7] The name of the test is glycohemoglobin, or glycosylated hemoglobin, or hemoglobin A1C, usually written HbA1C. The amount of hemoglobin A1C in the blood was measured so researchers could objectively compare blood sugar levels with the changes, if any, in eye or kidney health.

Advantages of Intensive Treatment

The patients in the group that had monthly medical visits and who took insulin at least three times a day (called the intensive management group) had the most normal hemoglobin A1C tests with the least deterioration in their medical condition over the nine years of the study. Even patients who had already shown some damage before the study began had a reduction in the damage by maintaining near-normal blood sugars. Intensive therapy reduced by 45 percent the risk of developing vision-threatening forms of retinopathy (disease of the retina of the eye) or retinopathy requiring laser treatment. Serious kidney disease was reduced by 56 percent, the occurrence of serious nerve disease was reduced by 60 per-

---

[6] Although the test has been available since the late 1970s, it is only now becoming widely used by physicians.

[7] Before this new test came along patients could fast for two days before a scheduled office visit so that their blood glucose laboratory result would indicate a normal value. Of course, this made the test useless but the patient avoided a big lecture from the doctor for being in poor control.

cent, and the risk of developing a high level of LDL (bad) cholesterol that could lead to strokes and heart attacks was also reduced.

To attain this almost normal blood sugar required a lot of extra work on the part of the patient and health care team. More frequent injections meant more frequent testing. The monthly visits with a physician or diabetes educators for any necessary adjustments of medication, diet, and other treatment elements were costly in time for both the patients and the medical team. In contrast, the group that received the standard treatment of one or two injections a day was seen four times a year by the health care team. The progression of diabetes complications in this standard therapy group was significantly higher.

So now there is *proof* that maintaining blood sugars in the normal range results in a decrease in the nerve and blood vessel damage that causes complications.

Disadvantages of Intensive Treatment

There is a downside to intensive treatment, however. First is the expense of taking more shots, testing more often, and consulting with doctors and other health care professionals more frequently.

Another disadvantage is the increased incidence of serious, unexpected low blood sugar events in intensive treatment. "Serious", means a low blood sugar that requires the help of another person because the person with diabetes is too impaired to get a glass of juice or eat glucose tablets. As mentioned above, some people who live alone or operate machinery would not be able to maintain a near-normal blood sugar if they experienced surprise lows as a side effect. However, although low blood sugar that needed help occurred more often, the average was only one additional serious low blood sugar event every two years.

The DCCT study puts to rest the debate about whether complications are a necessary consequence of diabetes. They are not. They are a result of high blood sugar. To the extent that high blood sugar can be prevented, a reduced incidence and reduced severity of complications will follow.

Doctors Weigh Several Factors Before Recommending Intensive Treatment

Do not expect, however, that every doctor will jump to change every diabetic patient's treatment plan. Some will want more proof; some will resist because they are so convinced that what they personally see in their practices is the truth; and some will feel that the costs in time and expense to their patients, especially their elderly patients, will not pay off.

Intensive Treatment For Older and Younger Folks

There are several advantages to intensively treating older adults even if they do not have a life expectancy of an additional 50 years. First, complications can begin appearing after only five years with the disease. Further, many people who are diagnosed in their middle years or later, have had it silently for several years with damage from high blood sugar already present. If we add the fact that the fastest-growing age group in this country is that of people over eighty-five, we can see that a sixty-five-year old newly diagnosed with diabetes may well live long enough to develop serious complications.

The strongest argument against intensive treatment for older adults is that low blood sugar can be dangerous, especially for people with hardening of the arteries. Strokes and heart attacks have been brought on by low blood sugar. However, if the patient is medically able and willing and can *safely* follow a strict treatment plan, the fact that he or she is sixty-five or seventy should not be the sole deterrent.

For children, especially those under two, intensive treatment, which attempts to keep blood sugar in the normal range, can be very risky. Since low blood sugar can impair normal brain development, which is not complete until seven years of age, it is safer to wait until the child is older and is better able to assist in intensive diabetes management. Until then, blood sugar is often allowed to remain a little on the high side.

Patients' Patience and Doctors' Patience

Yet another factor that influences how aggressive a doctor will get with a diabetes treatment program is how discouraged the physician is by patients' resisting medical advice. Patients (perhaps including your friend or family member) may believe that doctors see them only as people with diabetes, whereas patients see themselves first as mothers, employers, students, and basketball fans and, second, as people who happen to have diabetes. They commonly complain that their doctors want them to measure their food, check their blood sugar too frequently, exercise everyday, write everything down, and on and on. And sometimes their moms or some other important someone joins the doctor in the sermon titled "You have to take your diabetes seriously—it's important!"

And the person with diabetes says, "I know it's important, but, be real: I have a job. I have a life. I can't just do diabetes stuff all the time."

What is a doctor to do when he or she has just examined another patient who will lose a foot or whose kidneys have failed and will need dialysis, and whose next patient is one who won't follow doctor's orders? The consequences of sloppy diabetes management are very real to that doctor. However, to the patient they're only a remote possibility in the distant future.

Remember, most doctors chose medicine to help people. They can't help, however, if people won't come in for checkups because they think the doctor is too demanding. So maybe your friend's doctor doesn't even mention that exercise seven times a week is a good idea. If the patient says she's doing it three times a week on a good week, the doctor may give up with a "Do the best you can." Many good physicians have learned to walk a narrow line between urging what they know their patients should be doing and what they know the patient is willing to do.

The bottom line, though, is that the physician also knows that if the patient does not give time and attention to the inconvenient tasks of diabetes today, he or she may well pay with a lot more than inconvenience in a few years.

Intensive or Routine—Which Treatment Plan Does Your Friend or Family Member Have?

If doctors expect different things from their patients for many different reasons, what can you assume your friend or family member has been told by their doctor? Not much. They may have a doctor who is trying to keep their blood sugar normal or one who interferes minimally with the course of diabetes. The person with diabetes may also tell you something very different from what he or she heard in the doctor's office.

How You Can Help Your Relative or Friend Get the Best Treatment

Learn to Ask the Right Questions

If it's your responsibility to help manage your family member's diabetes treatment, you may have to learn the right questions to ask. This requires getting the kind of information this book and others have to offer. The "Suggested Reading" list in the Appendix is a good place to find out more.

At the rate that diabetes knowledge is growing, even a three-year-old book may be out-of-date. Don't ignore books, though. That would be like throwing the baby out with the bath water. Just don't make any decisions on treatment based on what could be old information. The three diabetes magazines listed under "Suggested Reading" are excellent sources on the latest in treatment and products (including foods).

Medicine is an imprecise science, so trying to determine if your loved one's doctor is doing the right thing is not easy. One way you can learn what is considered basic diabetes care by the American Diabetes Association is to send for their *Standards of Medical Care for Patients with Diabetes Mellitus*. This short guide was developed by 150 medical professionals experienced in diabetes treatment. The *Standards* outline and define what the physician should ask and check during the physical exam, what tests he or she should order, how often referrals should be made to eye and other specialists, how often return visits should be scheduled, and so forth.

A phrase that medical people sometimes hear is "That doctor orders a lot of tests just to pad the bill," Another is "Whenever you go to the doctor, he sends you to another one. They're all in cahoots to get a lot of money."

The Standards of Medical Care not only will allow you to assure yourself that everything is being done that should be done, it also will help you and your diabetic relative or friend understand why the doctor is recommending some tests and specialist consultations.

Certain tests are absolutely necessary to know what is happening with the kidneys and inside blood vessels and eyes. There is simply no way for your loved one to know if there is early or even moderate damage just by how he or she feels. Only a urine test, blood test, and thorough eye exam will answer the question "Is the treatment my dad or my sister getting the right treatment? Is a change called for?"

If your presence is welcome, go into the doctor's office with your family member or friend. Four ears are better than two. Together you will remember more of the doctor's instructions and comments and will be more likely to remember to ask all the questions you thought of on the way to the doctor's office. By the way, between appointments, write your questions out and insist on getting them all answered before you're ushered out.

Celeste, who's had diabetes for fourteen years, says, "No matter how silly you think the questions might be (they probably aren't, though), ask them, and make sure you fully understand the answers before you leave." Celeste's advice applies to you, as helper, too.

Another reason two listeners are better than one is that sometimes the patient hears only the diagnosis. The anxiety that comes with hearing the words *diabetes* or *kidney disease* can block out everything that the doctor says after that. And if the instructions sound like new information or

Sources for Diabetes Info

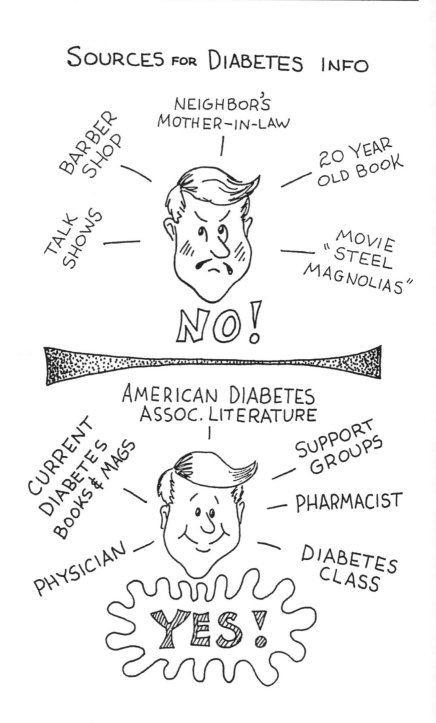

NEIGHBOR'S MOTHER-IN-LAW

BARBER SHOP

TALK SHOWS

20 YEAR OLD BOOK

MOVIE "STEEL MAGNOLIAS"

NO!

AMERICAN DIABETES ASSOC. LITERATURE

CURRENT DIABETES BOOKS & MAGS

SUPPORT GROUPS

PHARMACIST

PHYSICIAN

DIABETES CLASS

YES!

are complicated, ask the doctor to write them down. Or better yet, take a cassette recorder to the doctor's office and ask if you can record his or her comments and instructions. That way you won't miss a word.

If the doctor recommends some treatment that your friend or family member is afraid to follow, *be sure the doctor knows this.* One example is a fear of low blood sugar if insulin in increased. *The patient should leave the office convinced of the benefits of following the recommendation and armed with ways to prevent or handle any possible consequences.* For example, most low blood sugar episodes can be anticipated by more frequent blood glucose testing and by matching insulin to meals and exercise or vice versa.

Doctors with the best intentions may recommend changes that your family member or friend does not believe are possible. Quitting smoking, drinking, and/or losing weight are three hard changes to bring about and stay with. If the physician is made aware the patient probably cannot make such changes without more help, he or she will be able to recommend a supplemental program of smoking cessation, alcohol counselling, or weight control. If your special someone has tried self-control and it hasn't worked, it's time to try "Plan B" or some more creative alternative.

New medications and changes in medication can bring new situations. For those on oral medication, a frequent question is "What should I do if I forget to take my medicine?" Depending on the dosage and the medication, the doctor may say, "Take it now, even if it's two hours late" or "Take the next dose at the usual time." This is a good question to ask before you leave the office. You can also ask about possible side effects at this time, but there is another excellent source for this information—the pharmacist.

The Pharmacist Can Help

If you pick up medication for someone, ask the pharmacist about side effects; if the medicine should be taken before, with, or after a meal; if there is a generic form that is comparable (generic drugs are less expensive); if there's any medicine or food that is a bad combination with this medicine; if even small amounts of alcohol can cause a reaction; and if it's all right to drive after taking this medication. In fact, these are good questions to ask about any medicine—not just oral drugs to lower blood sugar. Many people are taking several medications, which may interact badly with each other.

The pharmacist can help anticipate problems with incompatible medicines. Nowadays, many pharmacies have computer files listing all customers' medications. These files can alert the pharmacist to problem combinations—*if* the customer buys all his or her medications at the same pharmacy or tells the pharmacist what else is being taken.

The Dentist and Periodontist

The same changes that occur in the blood vessels of the diabetic's eyes and other organs, can occur in the gums and the bone surrounding the teeth. And the reduced ability to fight infections can result in a greater chance of having mouth infections. One way the dentist has of suspecting that diabetes is not well-controlled, is if there are several gum abscesses or bone is being lost from around the teeth.

A long time diabetic has a greater risk of periodontal disease, the infection that destroys the bone around the teeth. It is a very common problem in *all* people, but it can be especially severe in someone with diabetes. It is also important to know that since gum problems are infections, they can make the management of the diabetes more difficult. So diabetes can make periodontal disease worse, and gum disease can make diabetes harder to control.

Some of the common signs of periodontal disease are bleeding gums, teeth that move out of position, multiple gum infections, partial dentures that don't fit well, and a bad taste or bad breath. A dentist is the person to see if you suspect a periodontal problem.

The good news is that if gums are healthy to begin with, and are *kept* that way, there is no reason to believe that the person with diabetes will have more problems than the non-diabetic.

Treatment Partners

Diabetes treatment is a team effort. The person with diabetes is really the most valuable player. Nothing anyone else on the team does can do much good if the star doesn't learn and practice good management.

Other team members can help a lot, though. They include the physician (preferably an endocrinologist), dietitian, nurse educator, exercise physiologist, counselor, podiatrist (foot specialist), pharmacist, and ophthalmologist.

The whole team won't always be necessary, but they do have special skills your friend or family member can use from time to time.

Don't forget that you too are a member of the team. Your help can keep your relative, colleague, or friend on track. Diabetes is too complex and too changeable to be a one-man or one-woman show.

Chapter 5

So Many Chores, So Little Time

What does someone with diabetes have to do to manage this condition? A lot. Just how much "a lot" is for your friend or family member depends on several things. Most important is whether they have Type I or Type II diabetes.

Why the Type of Diabetes is Important

The type of diabetes is very important in determining the treatment plan because people with Type I (insulin-dependent) diabetes generally have more erratic blood sugars, so they need to balance food, insulin, and exercise more precisely than someone with Type II diabetes. More careful balancing requires closer control of the amounts of carbohydrates eaten. It means timing meals to agree with insulin's peak action times. Since exercise can lower blood sugar, it means extra testing and perhaps extra food before, after, and sometimes during exercise. And since every insulin injection can influence blood sugar hours later, the timing of insulin, food, and exercise are crucial to her success at keeping blood sugar within a normal range.

Type I Diabetes

Chores For Those With Type I
Who Take Two Injections

Currently, most people with Type I diabetes are on a two-injection-per-day routine. This is what a typical day of diabetes chores is like for twenty-two year old Julie:

6:15 Examine feet after shower and apply foot lotion.
6:30 Check blood sugar before taking insulin.
6:33 Write result in log book.
6:35 Inject insulin (dosage may vary depending on blood sugar result so a chart may have to be consulted).
6:37 Write insulin dosage taken in log book.
7:05 Eat breakfast following prescribed meal plan.
— (Nothing diabetes-related until exercise or lunch).
12:00 Eat lunch following prescribed meal plan.

— (Nothing diabetes-related until exercise or dinner).

5:00 Check blood sugar before exercising.

5:03 Write result in log book.

5:05 Eat 1/2 sandwich because blood sugar was low
and will go down more with exercise.

5:10 Play tennis (not a very strenuous or long game so
don't need to stop midway to check blood sugar or snack).

5:45 Check blood sugar before taking insulin.

5:48 Write result in log book.

5:50 Inject insulin.

5:52 Write insulin dose taken in log book.

6:20 Eat dinner following prescribed meal plan.

9:30 Bedtime snack (crackers and milk).

— (Nothing diabetes-related until morning).

This plan is basic and involved only seventeen diabetes-related chores; chores that wouldn't be necessary if Julie's pancreas were working. But Julie has to "think" for her pancreas and supply the insulin at the appropriate time and in the right amounts. This schedule is for a routine day for Julie, without unusually high or low blood sugar. If she had had a high, she might have required a bigger dosage of insulin or even an extra injection.[1] A low might have meant eating extra food.

Checking Blood Sugar

Checking blood sugar and being able to make decisions based on the results is one of the most valuable advances in diabetes management. But testing is not done because it's easy or fun. It's done because nothing can take its place as a window into what's happening to blood sugar levels inside the body.

Getting that blood sugar reading is done either visually (without a meter) or automatically (with a meter).

Both methods require the person with diabetes to prick a finger to get a drop of blood onto a chemically treated strip. That's the part nobody likes. It hurts and can stay sore for a while.

---

[1] While an extra injection might seem an easy solution to every high blood sugar it is not usually recommended. It's too easy to take more than necessary and then get too low. Most people are told to increase the next day's dosage if there is a pattern of frequent highs at a particular time of day.

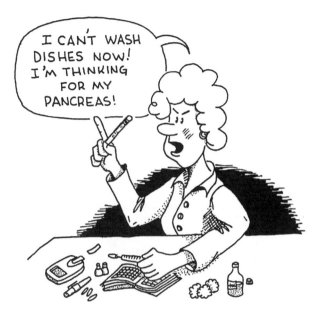

The Visual Method

If the visual method is used, that is, test strips without a meter, a finger is pricked with a lancet,[2] and a drop of blood is allowed to touch the strip. The blood drop on the strip is wiped off with a cotton ball after one minute, and after two minutes, the strip is held up to a color chart that has a number under each color. The closest-matching color is the approximate blood glucose level.[3] If the color of the strip is somewhere between two shades, an educated estimate is necessary. Trying to decide if the color of the strip is more like one color or the one above or below is a common source of irritation and some inaccuracy. If it really seems to be half-way

---

[2] A lancet is a single-pronged device used to prick a finger for a drop of blood. Most people load these into a pen-sized holder which requires just the push of a button to automatically spring-propel the lancet to the correct depth.

[3] The colors indicate a blood sugar range from 20 mg/dl to 800 mg/dl. In the lower values the difference between one block of color and the next higher one may be only 20 or 40, where small differences are more significant. The difference between the next to highest and the highest block jumps from 400 to 800.

between 120 and 180, for example, it's O.K. to average the two numbers and write down 150, but that's the limit of exactness possible. A recent study showed that subjects were five times more likely to *underestimate* a high of 240 which means they were less likely to recognize and acknowledge that some action should be taken. The same study also showed that people of all ages have difficulty reading the strips accurately.

Why do some people still do visual reading? Some like not carrying a meter and therefore use visual testing only when they are away from home. The more common reason, however is that it is much cheaper. Visual strips are one-half to one-third as expensive as the strips made for meters[4] and some users economize further by cutting them in half, which isn't possible when using a meter.

Using a Meter

A better method is to use a blood glucose meter to read the strip.[5] With a meter it is possible to get a more specific blood glucose level without guessing. The meter gives a relatively precise result and eliminates some of the steps (such as timing) that might be done incorrectly and cause an inaccurate and misleading test result. Mistakes are still possible—the most common is not getting a sufficiently big drop of blood on the strip. Doing all the steps from finger pricking to final result in front of a diabetes educator or physician can help spot mistakes in technique. In addition, accurate testing requires keeping the strips dry, running a test with a control solution[6] every week or so, and with some meters, regular cleaning.

Also, each meter has limitations and advantages. For example, some are particularly sensitive to temperature, so using them in a windy or drafty environment will give inaccurate results. Using a meter at high altitudes also requires some meter adjustments.

Knowing how to use the equipment correctly is still not enough. For testing to be an effective tool, the patient needs to know when and how often to test, and what to do with the results, besides just writing them down. Testing blood sugar provides vital feedback, which can help pro-

---

[4] Fifty visual strips are $10 to $18 (depending on the brand), while fifty meter strips usually run $30 to $32.

[5] A blood glucose meter is usually under $50 with the generous rebates manufacturers offer. The price of strips are the main cost factor, especially with several tests a day.

[6] Control solutions are made by every meter manufacturer to test that company's meter. Solutions are chemically prepared to give a known test range and should be periodically used instead of a drop of blood. If the meter reads outside of the range, either the meter or the strips are defective.

vide the motivation and basis to make adjustments in the treatment plan. Taking a larger dose of insulin, exercising (if blood sugar is high) or eating a larger bedtime snack (if blood sugar might get low in the middle of the night) are just three possibilities.

Most diabetics say blood testing is a nuisance, but they accept that it's as important as looking out their windshields when they're driving instead of at the pedals or at their passengers. How else can they know where they are and where they're going?

New Technology in Blood Glucose Meters

Researchers are trying to make blood sugar testing less painful and inconvenient. An implantable system has been developed that can give a blood sugar reading anytime a monitor is held near the area of the probe. The monitor is about one-third the size of a shoe box, small enough to be carried in a fanny pack or large handbag, but still not very handy. The developers estimate that another million dollars in research funds could make it the size of a wrist watch.

A different research group is working on a blood glucose tester that tests by analyzing light passing through a finger, rather like the red light you see through your hand when you hold the bright end of a flashlight in your palm. That monitor is still the size of two microwave ovens (the finger is placed between the two units). One optimistic estimate is that an improved model may be available for general use by 1999, and will cost about $1,500.

It's reassuring, though, to people with diabetes, that someday they may not have to prick their fingers and use drops of blood to test every time they want to know what their blood sugar is.

Keeping Records

People with diabetes usually write down anything that has an effect on their diabetes in a little diary, usually referred to as a log book. A log book is a valuable record of what the blood glucose results have been and when they've been high or low.

Besides the blood sugar results, people usually record the dosage and time they took their medication. They may also note any illness or stress, or a significant change in food ("Had a piece of cake at 3 P.M. party"). Some blood glucose meters have memories that record from one to 300 blood sugar results, some include the date and time of the test, and one model even allows the user to enter insulin dosages and other information.

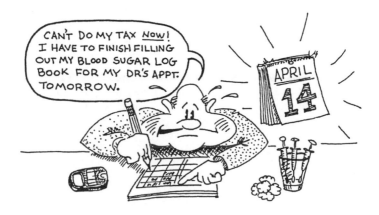

Some meters can be hooked up to computers that process results, even providing graphs to show blood sugar ups and downs. Having such results might make it easier for the diabetic to recognize patterns of blood sugar changes. It's also possible to rapidly send days of stored meter results over phone lines to the physician's office. There the physician or nurse specialist can assess the patterns and make changes in insulin that are more timely than was ever before possible when patients would just read off blood sugar values over the phone and all data had to be transcribed, compiled, and calculated by hand.

Experience and good record keeping, whether by sophisticated computer process or simple pencil and log book notations, tell the person and the doctor what, if any, changes need to be made in the time or dosage of medication.

Insulin Chores

The two-injections-a-day schedule wouldn't come close to keeping Julie's blood sugar under control if she only injected regular insulin. Regular insulin is active for only about four hours. Intermediate (NPH)[7] insulin is active for about twelve hours but wouldn't be able to handle the extra insulin needs of meals.

What Julie does is to mix regular and intermediate insulin together. And this is what most people do for at least one of their injections. The mixing process involves several steps:

---

[7] NPH stands for neutral protamine Hagedorn. Hagedorn was the scientist who developed a formula that extended the action of regular insulin by adding protamine.

Wipe tops of insulin bottles with alcohol.

Roll bottle of intermediate (NPH) insulin to gently mix.

Put air into syringe equal to the volume (units)[8] of NPH to be withdrawn.

Inject air into NPH bottle and remove needle and syringe.[9]

Put air into syringe equal to the amount of regular insulin to be withdrawn.

Inject air into regular insulin bottle and leave needle in bottle.

Turn the bottle of regular insulin upside down and pull plunger down to the amount of regular insulin to be taken.

Check syringe for air bubbles.[10] Flick syringe and squirt bubbles back into bottle, if present. Double-check that correct dosage has been drawn up, adjust if necessary, and remove needle and syringe.

Insert needle into NPH bottle.

Pull plunger down to the total amount of insulin to be given.

Remove needle and give injection in the subcutaneous tissue (the fatty layer just below the skin) of the abdomen, upper arm, thigh, or buttocks.

This description gives you an idea of just one of the skills (insulin mixing) that people who take insulin must learn.

By mixing the quick-acting insulin with intermediate insulin, it's possible to get almost the same benefit of four separate doses with only two shots.

The basic two-injection-a-day plan that is outlined above is the commonest treatment plan for an insulin-dependent diabetic but it isn't the only one.

Chores for Those Who Take Three or More Injections per Day

Many people who are insulin-dependent take insulin more frequently than Julie's two-injection schedule. The so-called intensive regimen of at least three injections a day attempts to more closely mimic a working pancreas by supplying insulin at every meal or at least at breakfast, dinner, and at bedtime. For most insulin-dependent diabetics, taking

---

[8] Insulin is measured in units instead of ounces or milligrams, as most medications are. There are 100 units in 1 cubic centimeter (cc). One cc is 1/30th of an ounce.

[9] An insulin bottle is air-tight so injecting air adds air pressure to help push the insulin out and into the syringe.

[10] Bubbles are air, not insulin, so bubbles mean the dosage of insulin in the syringe is less than prescribed.

three or four injections a day is the only way they can maintain *nearly normal* blood sugar.

Taking an injection before every meal means more blood glucose tests since a test is normally done before every injection to be sure the blood sugar is not too low. Another reason for testing before a shot may be to determine the insulin dosage. Unlike most medications that are taken one or more times a day in the same dosage, insulin needs may vary considerably, so many people are given a range of dosages from which to choose, depending on their blood sugar level.

This varying dosage plan, called a sliding scale, is not just for the person who takes three injections a day but also for those on an even more intensive treatment plan.

Here is one of the possible injection schedules for someone following an intensive treatment plan:

Before breakfast	Regular insulin
Before lunch	Regular insulin
Before dinner	Regular insulin
Before bedtime	Intermediate or long-acting insulin

A new very rapid-acting insulin Humalog (Lispro) has added more flexibility to treatment. Lispro starts acting within 5 minutes so it's possible to inject *after* a meal.

Whether the insulin is taken before the meal or after, a blood test is done before each of these injections. Many people also test two to three hours after meals to determine if they took the right amount of insulin. In addition, extra tests might be appropriate before, during, and after exercise and whenever extra monitoring is necessary, such as when the person is ill or the blood sugar is suspected to be too high or too low.

Blood testing is what makes an attempt at maintaining normal blood sugar possible.

Frequent injections and testing sound like a lot of work but they definitely pay off in the delay or prevention of diabetes complications. And there is another benefit, an immediate one. People taking an injection before every meal do not have to eat "by the clock." They don't need to take intermediate insulin at breakfast to take care of their lunch because they're planning on taking some regular insulin just before they eat lunch.

But Julie, who has only two injections a day, takes two types of insulin together, one to take care of breakfast, and the other for lunch–four to five hours *before* she eats lunch. This means her lunch time and the amount of food she will eat is written in stone. She might be able to go without a *good* lunch, but she'll have to drink milk, eat crackers, or eat or drink *something* that will keep her blood sugar from plummeting as the insulin she took five hours before is doing its "best" work.

People who have gotten over their initial aversion to the idea of taking four shots a day instead of the already distasteful two, generally love the freedom and flexibility it gives them.

The Insulin Pump

There is another way of taking insulin that tries to mimic a working pancreas but that doesn't require four injections a day. That is the insulin pump. The pump is a beeper-sized computer worn on a belt or in a pocket or bra. It holds an insulin-filled syringe or cartridge and measures out insulin through a tube and into the body.

Don has a pump. He had to learn how to use it, though, because it's very different from injections.

With the pump, Don still fills a syringe from an insulin bottle, but this is where the similarity ends. The syringe is a special one that fits into the pump, and instead of leaving the needle on the syringe, he takes it off. In the place of the needle, he attaches a piece of flexible tubing about the thickness of a strand of uncooked spaghetti and 24 to 42 inches long, depending on where he plans to insert it and how much length he needs. At the other end of the tubing, is a short needle that he inserts under his skin. He then tapes the needle down (In some cases, a flexible hollow piece of plastic can be used instead of a needle), pops the syringe into the pump case, and programs the pump to start pushing the plunger of the syringe. He tells the computer in the pump how much and when to push on the plunger.

Filling the syringe and fiddling with the tubing takes longer than an injection would, but Don only has to do this once every two or three days. The needle stays in place, and the syringe in the pump has enough insulin for three days of normal doses. There is also a brand of pump that uses insulin cartridges so no manual filling is needed.

Don programs the pump's computer to give him a basal rate, which is half of the total amount of insulin he takes a day spread over the entire twenty-four hours. The pump gives it to him a drop at a time which is much more like what the pancreas does.

Before a meal, Don checks his blood sugar, estimates how much he plans to eat, and programs the computer to give him a larger amount of insulin all at once, called a bolus. After the bolus is delivered, the pump returns to the basal rate and keeps giving him the tiny amount until he programs another change.

He can reduce the rate if he's going to exercise, or stop the pump if he wants to take it off to participate in contact or water sports or sexual relations. If he stays off the pump for more than two hours, he will probably have to take injections to compensate for not getting insulin from the pump.

Incidentally, not everyone removes the pump when they're being amorous. One young mother told me she just lays the pump next to her in bed—she does her thing and it does its.

The pump is not something that one buys at any drugstore or orders from a catalog. Don attended a couple of support groups of pump users to learn if he really wanted to take on this new challenge. His doctor wrote a letter to the insurance company to explain why the pump would be a better treatment than injections for Don. His doctor also wrote that she had confidence that Don would continue to test frequently and follow the safety practices the pump requires, such as changing the tubing at least every three days.

After the insurance company approved the expense, Don started his pump education.

He first had two classes with a dietitian to learn how to count carbohydrate grams. He already knew how to estimate the carbohydrate, protein, and fat in a portion size but carbohydrate counting is a more accurate way of matching food to insulin. He received charts and a book to help him calculate how much insulin he would need for the foods he ate at typical meals. He kept a food diary for a week and practiced. He called the dietitian when he had questions.

On the afternoon before he was to get the pump, Don came to the hospital outpatient diabetes center to get a demonstration model that had sterile water instead of insulin in the syringe. He was helped to insert the tubing for the first time. This rehearsal was to have him experience what it was like to sleep and shower at home with the pump.

The next morning before breakfast, he was admitted to the hospital for two days of hourly blood sugar testing and learning to use and adjust the pump's computer. The dietitian came in at every meal to check his skill in adding up grams of carbohydrate and setting the correct bolus amount. A nurse who was a specialist in diabetes education helped him learn how to change tubing, program the computer, and learn how to anticipate problems. Another part of Don's training was to use a treadmill in the cardiac rehabilitation department with an exercise physiologist who helped him analyze the effect exercise had on his blood sugar and to adjust the pump accordingly.

Don went home the second day with lots of practice under his belt. In some ways the pump was more work, but it freed him from having to eat on time or to eat the same amount of food and helped to reduce chances of complications.

Because of the frequent (four to eight times a day) blood glucose testing necessary to use the pump safely, it is not for someone who is "tired of doing all this diabetes stuff." It's true that Don doesn't give himself several separate injections, but more frequent testing, insertion of the needle, care of the tubing, filling of the insulin reservoir, and programming of the pump's computer all make for anything but a lazy way of managing the taking of insulin.

The insulin pump uses only regular, quick-acting insulin, which has good and bad aspects. The good news is that if the blood sugar is too high or too low, the computer can be directed to increase or decrease the amount of insulin released, and it will work quickly. Unlike intermediate or long-acting insulin which, once injected, can't be cut back or prevented from being absorbed for many hours, regular insulin has a short life; if too much goes in, it quickly wears off, so it requires less increase in food. And, if more insulin is needed, a pump user just presses a few buttons on the computer. Anyone else has to get out the insulin vial, syringe, swab, and find a place to take an extra injection.

The bad aspect of the pump is also due to the regular insulin it uses. The short life of regular insulin means that if anything causes an interruption in the flow, blood sugar will quickly climb. There is no back-up of intermediate insulin taken hours before that will, at least partly, control sugar levels, as would be the case with using mixed insulins for a standard two-injection schedule. An interruption can be caused by a kink in the tubing, a clog in the needle under the skin, an infection or allergy where the needle is placed that interferes with absorption, or a battery failure.

Another way pump users (or any insulin user, really) can fail to get the insulin they need is when the insulin "fries." One young woman told me her blood sugar started going up after a trip to the beach. She changed her tubing and checked her battery but her sugar level still didn't come down. The last thing she tried was changing the insulin in the reservoir of the pump, and that worked. It turned out her insulin had gotten overheated next to her in the sun and had become ineffective.[11] If she had not discovered the cause of the pump problem on her own, however, she wouldn't have been in danger. She would have called her physician for instructions and gone back to taking her previous insulin dosage by injection until the pump problem was solved.

---

[11] Insulin doesn't have to be kept refrigerated but it can't be kept at over 100 degrees F. for an extended period.

In all the above causes of pump failure, except for actually discovering that the needle has come out, it is the blood sugar level that will alert the user that something needs adjustment. Again, pumps are for the conscientious tester, not the poorly motivated.

Who Pays For The Insulin Pump

The pump has one other big disadvantage—it's very expensive. The pump itself costs about $4,000 to $5,000, and supplies (tubing, etc.) run about $120 per month. In addition, there is usually a hospital stay of two or three days while a new user like Don is trained and monitored, plus two or three outpatient classes. Some insurance companies will pay 80 percent of the initial cost and supplies, but they usually must be convinced that it will be worth the outlay by preventing expensive hospitalizations for complications that would probably occur or get worse if the candidate did not have a pump. Convincing an insurance company of the cost-effectiveness of the pump for a particular person usually means that the physician has to write letters and make phone calls spelling out the medical benefits of pump therapy to the patient and the financial benefits to the insurance company.

Although Don wanted the pump to add more flexibility to his lifestyle, he and his physician had a more serious reason that convinced the insurance company it would be cheaper to pay for a pump now than complications later. Don's last eye checkup showed some unfavorable changes in the retina of his eye. Eighteen years with diabetes were taking their toll. Don, his doctor, and the insurance company wanted to prevent progression of eye disease. The best way of accomplishing that goal was to keep his blood sugar as close to normal as possible.

So Don got his pump, and with it a better tool to delay, and maybe prevent, complications.

Eating Can Be A Chore

Since everybody has to eat, it may not seem that meals and snacks should be counted as diabetes-related chores. The reason that they are included here is that meals are neither flexible in amount nor optional, as they are for most of us. Consistency is the key word. Meals are scheduled, mandatory, and demand mental calculations like "Is the amount of carbohydrate in my prescribed diet the same as the amount in this serving?"

The necessity to eat a certain amount and to eat it on time is a considerable nuisance. Julie, and most people with Type I diabetes I talked with, listed it as one of the top ten diabetes "pains in the neck." Eating on schedule means Julie may have to eat when she isn't hungry. Or maybe she doesn't want to eat because she's concentrating intensely on some interesting school or work project. No matter. She *must* stop and eat. That means, too, that she must carry food wherever she goes. At the very least she must carry some form of fast-acting sugar like glucose tablets or hard candies.

It also means that she cannot easily sleep in on Sunday morning because she needs to take her insulin (whose effect has worn off from the pre-dinner injection of last night). But she can't take her insulin without eating thirty minutes later. So the morning she wants to sleep in is really a morning she tests her blood sugar, logs the results, takes her injection, waits thirty minutes to eat, eats breakfast, and *then* goes back to bed for her well-deserved "slothfest."

Being Prepared for Every Situation

As "simple" as Julie's schedule is (there's no insulin injection before lunch), most people still carry their insulin and meter with them in case of some change in plans. That means a kit with the following supplies:

> Regular insulin
> Intermediate insulin
> Syringe(s)
> Alcohol swabs
> Blood glucose strips
> Blood glucose meter
> Lancet device to get drop of blood
> Spare lancets
> Cotton balls or tissue
> Log book to record results and
>   pencil or pen

And you think *your* handbag, backpack, or briefcase is crowded! How about adding all of the above plus your emergency candy, food, or juice?

There are some space-saving devices that can help a bit with the paraphernalia load. One of these is an insulin pen that holds a cartridge of insulin in a self-contained holder and needle. It eliminates the need for a vial of insulin-the syringe and vial are all incorporated into one device.

Another space saver is the blood glucose meter with a memory. Many of these allow the user to do scores of blood glucose tests and recall them with the push of a button. Julie's doesn't have a way to record the dosage of insulin she gave herself, though, so she still has to write *something* down. Still, the memory means she can wait to write down the results of the day's blood sugar tests until she's at home at the kitchen table—sort of like balancing your checkbook at home when you feel like it instead of while standing at the cashier's counter after every transaction.

The bottom line, though, is that she's got to carry stuff and it's not stuff than anybody else has to bother with. It's not a *huge* pain, but it is another irritation that having diabetes brings.

Foot Care

Foot care is important for everyone with diabetes. Feet can lose sensation when high blood sugar damages nerves. It's possible to have a deep sore, cut, or a nasty infection and not feel a twinge.

Diabetics are urged to let their eyes tell them if there is a problem. Julie checks her feet every day after her shower. She looks for white or reddened areas,[12] blisters, ingrown toenails, and athlete's foot. She applies a special lotion to her feet to keep them from getting dry and cracked because cracks can be an entry point for infection-causing germs.

There are many things Julie *doesn't* do because she has diabetes. She doesn't walk around barefoot or in open-toed shoes or sandals, and she doesn't use corn plasters or chemicals to remove corns or callouses. She certainly doesn't do "bathroom surgery" such as using razor blades to remove corns; a podiatrist does that for her.

One more thing Julie doesn't do is soak her feet. I know, people used to think a nice, long soak in Epsom salts was good for feet. Well, it isn't good for diabetic feet! There are several reasons for this. First, with poor nerve sensation, too many people have burned themselves in water that was really too hot but felt just fine to them. Even if Julie avoids that danger by using a thermometer, there's another problem. Although her feet would feel moisturized when she pulled them out of the water, the long-term effect of soaking is drying. Soaking removes the natural oils that no amount of lotion can totally replace, thereby making her skin drier and more prone to cracks and infections than before.

The last reason why soaking is not advised is that warmth to a body part increases the metabolism of the cells in that area. Usually that is no problem. The blood vessels in the area dilate and more blood comes in with the additional food and oxygen required by the increased metabolism. But what if the blood vessels are narrowed by fatty deposits or rigid walls? In that case, the extra blood won't be able to get to the cells

---

[12] Red areas may indicate an infection near the surface. Whitened areas indicate an infection deeper inside the tissue.

and they will suffer from insufficient oxygen and glucose. Some will even die. Hot soaks, hot water bottles, and hot pads should be avoided by people with diabetes. So don't buy any electric foot soakers as a present for someone with diabetes. Offer a gentle foot massage with lotion. We all like massages.

You may be able to help with some aspects of foot care if you live with a person with diabetes. If they have poor vision or are not very flexible and can't see all parts of their feet you could be the "foot checker."

If you go with the diabetic to the doctor's office, remind him or her to take off shoes and socks before the doctor comes in. Busy physicians can forget feet when they're checking heart, lungs, and blood pressure. Exposed feet get their attention.

Type II Diabetes

Some people with diabetes still have some functioning insulin-producing cells and do not need insulin as part of their treatment. For these people, exercise and diet alone may maintain blood sugar within normal limits. For some, oral medication that lowers blood sugar may also be needed.

Oral Diabetes Medication

Oral diabetes medications are *not* a pill form of insulin. They are not effective if there are no insulin-producing cells in the pancreas. Although these drugs can't replace insulin, and are unlikely to be effective if the diet is ignored, they do have one or more of these helpful effects:

1. They stimulate the pancreas to release insulin.
2. They help insulin bind to the cell so glucose can enter.
3. They may increase the number of insulin receptor sites on cells.
4. They may suppress the release of glucose from the liver.
5. They may slow down the absorption of table sugars from the digestive system.

The result is that more insulin is available or is more effective, so more sugar is able to leave the blood and get into the cells. That means the blood sugar will go down, and without attention, it could go down too far.

Preventing Blood Sugar from Going Too Low

Low blood sugar can be dangerous or even fatal, so a person who is taking blood sugar lowering pills has to take some precautions, just as insulin users do.

Precautions to prevent low blood sugar include:

Not having more than 1 or 2 alcoholic drinks;
Not drinking alcoholic drinks without a meal;
Not eating later than usual;
Not skipping meals;
Not eating less than the amount calculated by the physician or dietitian to match the effect of the medicine.

These precautions mean that eating on schedule is important for those on some oral medications. The low blood sugar that can occur as a consequence of not taking in enough food can be severe and prolonged. The severity varies with the person's condition and time without food. Most pills are meant to be effective for 12 to 24 hours, so a low blood sugar level can last a long time.

Checking Blood Sugar

Because people who take oral medication have some insulin production and a less impaired ability to regulate their blood sugar, they tend to have less erratic swings in blood sugar levels than someone who is dependent on injected insulin. This means it usually is not necessary for them to check their blood sugar as often.

Physicians have many different opinions about when and how often blood sugar needs to be checked by someone with Type II diabetes who does not require insulin. Recommendations range from twice a week to four times a day. Some doctors ask their patients to check once a day before breakfast. Others have them check before breakfast and dinner when they usually take their pill. While some patients are learning to balance their exercise, diet, and medication, they may need to test as often as a person taking insulin. Or they may test an hour or two *after* meals to check what effect the foods they just ate have on their blood sugar level. Some patients find they have very stable blood glucose levels when they stay on their diet, exercise, and medication program, so their doctors recommend decreasing blood glucose testing to twice a week. Unfortunately, sometimes the deciding factor in how often blood sugar testing is performed is the cost of the strips, not the medical necessity.

Why Insulin May Be Necessary

Type II diabetes frequently progresses in severity over the years, so different treatments may be needed at different times. Diet, weight loss, and regular exercise are usually tried first. Next, the doctor will usually prescribe oral medication. If oral medication at the maximum dosage doesn't work, insulin must be injected.

Many people resist taking insulin for several reasons. First, they may believe it is a punishment from the doctor for their inability to lose excess weight and keep it off. They may have had good results from oral medication for years. It may have been necessary for the doctor to increase the dosage from time to time to keep their blood sugar within normal limits, but most patients accept taking a few more pills as a minor inconvenience and expense.

The trouble comes when the patient is taking the maximum dosage of the medicine and the doctors says, "The pills aren't working. We'll have to go to insulin."

The patient's response frequently is, "Well, they worked in the past and all you did was prescribe more pills, so do it again."

The problem is that exceeding the maximum dosage won't work. The situation is similar to your taking aspirin for a headache. Just because two tablets work for your usual headache, taking twenty won't relieve the agony of a migraine. No amount of aspirin would be effective for that degree of pain, and taking twenty tablets would be toxic besides. More is not always better.

Not everyone with Type II diabetes moves from diet, weight loss, and exercise to oral medication and eventually to insulin. Many times, if the patient can lose weight, no medication is necessary. Or maybe the oral medication is only necessary in the beginning to get the high blood sugar under control while the person gets a diet and exercise program going.

Or the person may get the flu or be hospitalized for some nondiabetes-related condition or surgery and need insulin to handle the stress. In such a case, the diabetic could be back on just diet and exercise in a matter of a few weeks.

Insulin-Dependent or Insulin-Requiring?

I'd like to straighten out a common misunderstanding about the difference between Type I and Type II diabetes. You know by now that all people with Type I diabetes *must* take insulin. Another description for their condition is *insulin-dependent* diabetes.

But many people with Type II diabetes who eventually must take insulin believe that they have become transformed into Type I diabetics. This is almost never the case. They have become insulin-*requiring* but are not insulin-*dependent*. There is a difference. They need some insulin to keep their blood sugar in the normal range, but without it they would live for months and even years. They'd feel unwell, and they'd develop complications faster than if their blood sugar were within normal limits. If they got an infection, they might develop dangerously high blood sugar and become dehydrated. But without insulin they wouldn't necessarily die in a few days or weeks. That's the difference. A person with Type I diabetes will die in a short time without insulin.

Chores for Someone with Type II Diabetes

Chores of the person with Type II diabetes include a variety of things they might or might not need to do. Here are the recommended chores for good diabetes management of Type II diabetes:

1. Exercise 3 to 7 times a week.
2. Check feet daily.
3. Avoid concentrated sweets.
4. Lose weight or maintain ideal body weight.
5. Test blood sugar 2 to 28 times a week.
6. Eat meals on time in required amounts.
7. Take oral medication (maybe).
8. Take insulin (maybe).

The good news about Type II diabetes is that blood sugar control is not as difficult as with Type I. Usually diet and testing are less rigorous. And insulin is a "maybe," not a requirement.

The bad news is that if Type II diabetes is not taken seriously, if the recommended chores are not done, the same complications that can happen to someone with Type I diabetes, can happen to someone with Type II.

Shared Attitudes About Chores With Both Types of Diabetes

The chores of diabetes are many. Here's what it adds up to after twenty years for someone taking only two shots a day, checking blood glucose three times a day, exercising and checking feet once a day, seeing the doctor who takes care of their diabetes every three months, an eye doctor once a year, and reading one diabetes magazine once a month:

Diabetes magazine	240 issues
Eye doctor	20 visits
Diabetes doctor	80 visits
Exercise	7300 times
Foot checks	7300 times
Blood sugar	21,900 tests
Insulin	14,600 shots

And the chores never end. Neither can they be put aside like the ironing or washing the car until the person "feels like it."

Not everyone with diabetes sees the chores as a terrible burden. Some have accepted them as a normal part of their lives like brushing and flossing their teeth. My hat is off to them.

For your friend, family member, or colleague, it may not be possible yet to take these chores in stride. They may see them as painful and inconvenient reminders of their diabetes and its scary complications.

You can help by listening to the gripes. It *isn't* fair that they have diabetes to deal with every day. Eventually, they may share Celeste's attitude. She says, "I have a lot to be thankful for, and take things a day at a time so that I know my future will be the best I can make it."

Chapter 6
Diabetes - A Pain in the Wallet

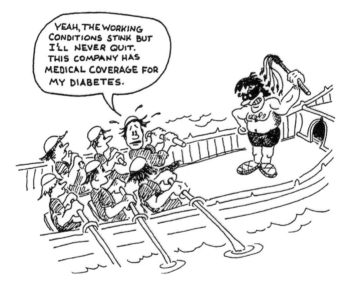

YEAH, THE WORKING CONDITIONS STINK BUT I'LL NEVER QUIT. THIS COMPANY HAS MEDICAL COVERAGE FOR MY DIABETES.

Sherill was in a no-win situation. She had a job, health insurance, and diabetes. Her husband didn't have diabetes, but he didn't have a job, either. Four months ago the company he worked for went bankrupt. He applied to dozens of companies in the city where they lived, but nothing materialized. Through contacts, he finally got a job offer in another state. The family had to make a hard choice.

Sherill could keep her job with its insurance and they could get further in debt living on her salary while her husband kept looking for work in their area. Or her husband could take the out-of-state job, she could quit hers, and they could sign up for insurance at her husband's new company. *But,* that insurance would not cover any diabetes-related problem for a year or two because her diabetes is a pre-existing condition. During this period, if Sherill had any health condition that could possibly be attributed to diabetes, she and her husband would have to pay for it out of their own pockets. They could lose all their savings, the equity in their house, and even wind up in debt if she required an operation, or a week or two in the hospital. This is the kind of problem people with diabetes face every day. Switching jobs is a big risk for them if it means changing insurance carriers. Fortunately, a new law has lessened that risk. The Health Insurance Portability and Accountability Act of 1996, seeks to improve the availability of health insurance and make it easier to move from one source of health insurance to another without restrictions for pre-existing health conditions. The effectiveness of this law depends on a number of variables including origin and destination employers' health benefit rules, and relevant state(s)' laws.

No Job—No Insurance

Switching jobs or getting a pink slip is not the only way to lose insurance. Many companies stop covering dependents when they reach twenty-one. Adult sons or daughters have to find their own insurance or the family has to find a more expensive plan that will accept the "dependent."

A twenty-nine year old woman told me her parents pay $744 a month for insurance that includes her. She said, "I'm so scared of what will happen when they can't pay it anymore—I sure can't."

Diabetes can have enormous impact on career choice. Many young people with diabetes are counseled to prepare for the day they are no longer on their parents' policy by seeking and keeping a job with the government or some other employer that offers a group policy with comprehensive health benefits. Federal, state, and municipal governments and large corporations have traditionally been havens for people with health conditions or who have family members with chronic problems. Keeping that job can be more important than liking the work. Who would dare leave a job with a company that provided even halfway-generous health insurance and opt for the insecurity of Sherill and her family's situation?

Being self-employed or employed in a small service business is not a luxury most people with diabetes can afford. They've discovered that many small businesses can't afford to keep them when the bill for health insurance comes back doubled or tripled because of one employee with cancer, heart disease, or diabetes.

If the employer can't or won't pay for insurance coverage, that leaves the option of getting an individual policy. If you can find one. Virtually no private insurance companies and only a handful of Blue Cross and Blue Shield plans will sell policies to individuals with diabetes. Getting insurance through a big company may be the only way to get coverage. Twenty-three states have a high-risk insurance pool for people who can't get insurance. It doesn't always come cheap, though. Some premiums are $1,000 a month with a $5,000 deductible.

Getting Hired or Fired

One of the hurdles to getting the insurance is getting the job in the first place. One recent study showed that when job applicants disclosed they had diabetes in a job interview, they were turned down two and a half times more often than their brothers or sisters without diabetes. If they didn't tell the interviewer they had diabetes, they had no more chance of being refused a job than their siblings.

Even if a diabetic makes it past the interview, there may still be a company physician with outmoded ideas of what a person with diabetes can and can't do. In truth, workers with no diabetic complications have no higher absenteeism rates than workers without diabetes.

There is no requirement that a person volunteer information to employers or insurance companies about diabetes or any other medical condition. But once the person has "confessed" to one insurance company and is refused, or files a claim for a hospitalization, the information will be recorded at the Medical Information Bureau, an industry clearinghouse. This big computer system will likely be consulted by any insurance companies that get that person's application from then on.

If one decides to disclose his/her diabetes, it probably would be very helpful to include as many positive aspects as posible, including the considerable loyalty such an employee feels toward an employer, the discipline in life that carries over to one's duties at work, the manageability of the employee's condition...

The Americans With Disabilities Act, and the Family and Medical Leave Act provide, or at least intend to provide, subtantial protection to, among others, folks with diabetes with respect to hiring, firing, and accommodation on the job.

The problems with these laws are that since they are new or enforcement has only recently commenced, the number of high level court cases that have ruled on their different aspects are relatively limited. One's rights are not yet clearly defined.

So while a person with diabetes or other chronic health problem may be *theoretically* protected, an employer may *assert* another reason for teminating or not hiring an employee, while his/her real motivation for action is the diabetes, asthma, etc.

Unfortunately there is still good reason to be cautious

The Medicare Maze

Most people over sixty-five and those with severe complications such as kidney failure, blindness or amputations, have Medicare, which is a great help but still doesn't pay all the costs.

After figuring the approved charge, deductible, fee cap, and co-payment, Medicare usually pays about half of the cost of medical treatment. The remainder must be paid by the patient or by supplemental insurance.

There are many supplies and treatments that Medicare does not pay for. The following is not a complete list of what is and is not reimbursed to the person with diabetes, but it demonstrates an interesting pattern: the items that *prevent* serious and expensive problems are primarily on the "Medicare Doesn't Pay" side of the list. The exceptions are theraputic shoes, minimal routine foot care, and meters and home blood glucose testing supplies *for those taking insulin*. Blood glucose testing, however, should be done by everyone with diabetes, even if he or she is not using insulin. If testing is not done, or not done frequently enough because the person can't afford the strips and lancets, the blood sugar level can only be guessed at. Consequently, blood sugar control may suffer and costly complications may result.

Medicare Doesn't Pay For:	Medicare Pays For:
Diabetes education	Diabetic foot care &
Insulin	therapeutic shoes
Syringes	Kidney dialysis
Blood glucose meters and	Blood glucose meters and
testing supplies of	test strips for insulin users
non-insulin users	Hyperbaric chamber treatment[1]
Insulin pumps	Wheelchairs
Routine eye exams	Artificial limbs
Eyeglasses	Laser treatments for
Oral medication	retinopathy
Dietetic foods	Corrective lenses after
	cataract surgery
	Special equipment for the
	visually impaired

Currently, Congress is considering adding blood glucose strips coverage regardless of insulin need and diabetes education to medicare benefits. These Medicare changes would save hundreds of millions of dollars every year in expensive treatment and hospializations for complications and prevent untold suffering.

What If Your Relative or Friend Doesn't Have Medicare?

What Medicare covers is important to every person with diabetes because Health Maintenance Organizations (HMOs) such as Kaiser

---

[1] A hyperbaric chamber is an airtight room or chamber that administers oxygen under pressure. Increased oxygen concentration in tissues helps in healing diabetic ulcers, gangrene, and other serious infections. It was originally, and still is, used to treat "the bends" in divers.

Permanente and Cigna, private insurance companies, and self-insured companies frequently adopt Medicare guidelines as their own.[2] What Medicare is willing to pay for often becomes the industry standard; what it refuses to cover is felt to be appropriate for others to refuse too.

Experimental Procedures

The Medicare policy of not paying for procedures it has labeled "experimental" or "investigational" means that the $4,000 purchase price of an insulin pump that could facilitate maintenance of near-normal blood sugar is not covered by Medicare, and only sometimes by insurance companies. The pump has been shown to slow the progress of kidney and eye disease in users and to prevent congenital defects in the newborns of diabetic mothers with pumps. If a physician writes a detailed letter explaining that specific patient's need for a pump, that patient may eventually get 80 percent of the cost of the pump covered. The doctor's effort solves that particular patient's problem but does little to *change our national practice of paying for treatment of complications instead of their prevention.* The annual cost of kidney dialysis for one patient (not counting physician visits, transportation, or medication) is about $30,000. Shouldn't we be preventing this misery and expense by being willing to pay for *thorough, early* diabetes care?

A pancreas transplant, the only cure for diabetes,[3] is even less frequently covered by insurance. The government insurance company for the dependents of members of the armed forces, CHAMPUS, joins Medicare in refusing to pay for this procedure despite its twenty-seven-year existence and a current 50 to 70 percent five-year success rate.[4] Most insurance companies are as reluctant as CHAMPUS to cover pancreas transplants because of the expense. Since a pancreas transplant costs about $150,000, this means almost no one can afford the only cure for diabetes. It also means that the operation is done only when the patient already has complications, when he or she is desperate and can make a good case that he or she will die from a complication in a short time if the transplant is not approved. Unfortunately, if the transplant had been done years earlier those complications could have been prevented.

At this time, escalating medical costs leading to insurance cut-backs and the allocation of funds to other conditions mean doors of hope are closed to many with diabetes.

---

[2] Self-insured companies establish a fund for employee health expenses instead of paying an insurance company premiums. Frequently they contract with an insurance company to review claims but the decision of what to pay for is their own.

Supplies and Physician Fees

Even if the person with diabetes never needs a transplant or kidney dialysis, he or she will have other substantial expenses.

Since diabetes management ranges from no medication and no testing to testing eight times a day and use of an insulin pump, the monthly cost of supplies also varies. Another variable, of course, is what is reimbursed and what is not. Personal out-of-pocket expenses for supplies can range from zero to over $200 a month.

Test strips for testing blood at home are 60 to 70 cents each. Multiply that by four to eight tests a day, and you have a monthly budget item of around $70 to $150 just for test strips!

In addition to strips, supplies include insulin, oral medication, lancet device and lancets, syringes, approved containers for used needles and lancets, alcohol swabs, foot creams, glucose tablets, ketone strips, and meter control solution.

Not included in the above list are less frequently bought items such as meters and batteries, traveling cases for supplies, diabetes identification bracelets, books (including cookbooks), and diabetes magazine subscriptions.

Physician fees and laboratory bills also vary widely. Many people have Medicare or HMOs that pay ninety to one hundred percent of physician fees. Others pay for all office visits from their own pockets-the range is considerable. Your friend or relative may have excellent coverage. I hope so, because if not, he or she may wait for a problem to become serious, or forego regular checkups and tests because office visits for preventive care are just not affordable.

An office visit to a general practitioner runs $40 to $60, and lab test fees are about $150. Multiply those figures by the two, three, or four routine visits a year that are recommended for diabetes patients in good control, and you get an annual cost of $380 to $840. Someone whose diabetes is out of control or who has some complication will need more frequent visits and lab tests, and possibly outpatient treatment or hospitalization.

In addition to a general practitioner, some patients see a diabetes specialist whose fee may be $125 or more for the first consultation. Follow-up visits run closer to $60 each.

An annual visit to an eye specialist is also a must to catch problems while they are still treatable. Eye exams can cost up to $200 but the average is 50 to 120 dollars.

[3] Some patients who have had pancreas transplants that eventually failed have related that despite the discomfort, danger, and expense of the operation and recovery, the months of no diabetes while the graft was functioning were so wonderful, they would do it again. Those who have the financial resources are usually willing to undergo a second transplant.
[4] A 50-70% five-year success rate refers to how often the new pancreas was not rejected during that time. The patient *survival* rate is actually 90% for one year after surgery.

Dentist visits may need to be more frequent because of gum disease which is more prevalent with diabetes.

Another health practitioner that diabetics see more often than the general public is a podiatrist. This foot specialist prevents, diagnoses, and treats foot problems.

Fees for these health care providers may be higher or lower in different parts of the country, and sometimes insurance pays part of these expenses, but many times, whatever the fees, they're the patient's burden alone.

Even food can be more expensive. Fresh fruits and vegetables, low-fat meats, artificial sweeteners, fat substitutes, and dietetic foods can all add to the cost of diabetes.

It Doesn't Always Make Sense

As we saw in the earlier section on Medicare, private insurance may pay for some of the supplies, but what they'll pay for and what they refuse to cover make no sense. For example, one woman told me that her company pays for the insulin, but not the syringes to inject it!

There are over 1,000 private insurance companies in the United States, each with different rules and different forms. The mass and complexity of the paperwork necessary to get what one is entitled to, has created a new industry of claims collectors who fill out insurance forms, intercede with the insurance company when necessary, and make sure the customer receives his due. It's no wonder that twenty-four percent of health care costs in the United States go to pay for administrative expense.

The very irrationality of the payment issue creates ongoing frustration and not infrequent laments, such as Sherill's "I feel like I have two diseases, diabetes and insuranceitis."

Insurance and Education

Most insurance plans have acknowledged that people with diabetes can benefit from some education in learning about the condition. Unfortunately, this too often is lip service. Most insurance carriers cover only $120 worth of diabetes education for the patient's lifetime! Considering that the average basic eight-hour group diabetes course costs twice that, it makes you wonder how genuinely education is valued. Consider too, that needs change over time. Someone who was diagnosed twenty years ago may need to be up-dated on blood sugar testing or may need to start a more intensive program that requires learning more about adjusting insulin and fine-tuning diet. Someone with Type II diabetes who has been taking pills for years, may now need insulin instruction and the diet changes necessary to get insulin and food in sync. What is that person to do if the $120 was spent when he or she was first diagnosed? Is a five-minute mini-class with a nurse in the physician's office enough? Are pamphlets going to do the job? Diabetes educators bemoan the fact that their hands are tied by unrealistic limitations.

It Can Get Crazy!

As if the insurance maze, cost of supplies, and need to choose one's employment based on diabetes demands were not enough, another problem can come from the expense of diabetes not being recognized. A seventeen year old young man from South Carolina told me that he has been turned down for student loans because his parents' income is a little too high for him to qualify. In his family money is fairly tight, when you consider that he has to spend at least $175 per month on diabetes supplies alone. If just that annual $2,100 cost were subtracted from his father's income, he would qualify for a student loan. He wishes someone would take his unavoidable medical expenses into consideration when computing his loan eligibility.

Pay the Doctor or Pay the Rent?

The downside of all these expenses is that good diabetes management can get sacrificed to cut costs. The first economy usually is less frequent blood sugar testing since buying strips adds up so quickly. Next are fewer doctor visits or skipping the annual eye exam. Missing check-ups economizes not only on the doctor's fee but on lab test fees too. However, it can also mean not finding a condition while it is still treatable.

No study has shown that reimbursing for supplies automatically improves diabetes control, but many studies have shown that what is *not* reimbursed is less frequently purchased and used.

Whatever your feelings on whether publicly funded medical benefits should be raised or lowered, it's clear that the present setup is irrational. It makes no sense to refuse payment for preventive treatment but pay for acute care and allow permanently disabling complications that cost orders of magnitude more.

Without a saner health policy, people with diabetes will frequently be forced to choose between affording good preventive care and providing necessities for themselves and their families. Such a compromise can cost them and all of us dearly.

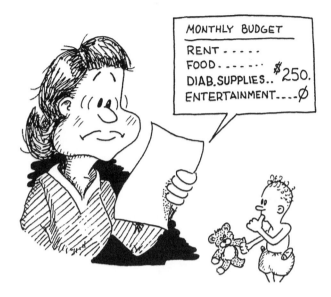

How You Can Help

Dealing with the health care system may seem like something you can't tackle but there are some very important ways in which you can help:

1. You can telephone insurance companies for a friend, colleague, or relative who is shopping for coverage. Find out premiums, deductibles, and what's covered. This way you will be a buffer and can spare the person with diabetes (if he or she wants to be spared) from hearing bad news. You can pass along only what is useful.

For people who have been refused insurance because of their diabetes, an insurance risk pool may be the answer. For a sometimes modest premium the person receives insurance coverage. The insurance companies operating in the state divide up the difference between the amount collected in premiums and the actual amount spent for health care services to the members in the pool. Twenty-six states have, or are considering establishing, state risk pools. To find out if your state has such a pool, look in the state government offices section of the white pages of your phone book, perhaps under "Health Division."

2. Giving help in getting insurance reimbursement can be a wonderful gift. It's not only filling out the forms that's a chore, but collecting receipts, talking with physicians and laboratory billing personnel, and defending your relative or friend's need to the insurance company. Many times a third person can be a better advocate than the insured.

3. If your friend or relative is shopping for a new physician, join the search. Ask any health care workers you know for recommendations of whom they would go to if they had diabetes. Call physicians' offices and find out the cost of a visit and the policy on "accepting assignment" (taking as payment in full whatever the insurance company or Medicare pays). Also ask about spreading out payments for services. These chores can sometimes seem overwhelming. They may make the diabetic postpone getting care rather than have to deal with embarrassing money details.

4. Ask if you can help in other concrete ways. If you suspect a gift of diabetes supplies would be welcome, ask. Perhaps the person living on a fixed income would appreciate a box of strips instead of another slip or bottle of aftershave next Christmas.

5. Last, but certainly not least, write and call your congressmen and congresswomen when legislation affecting diabetes research, treatment, or health care system changes is being considered. And get your whole network of friends and relatives to join you. Some sources say that every letter that is received counts as four hundred who share your view but didn't write.

There's a lot you can do directly for your relative, friend, or colleague. And there are opportunities to make things better for people with diabetes in general, too. You can do well by doing good.

Chapter 7
Complications Go from Head to Toe

Robert was forty-three years old and had a huge infected sore on his foot when he was admitted to our hospital. He had had a small blister on his foot the previous morning but had gone to his work as a cook, standing and walking all day as usual. That evening, when he removed his shoe, he was horrified to discover that the tiny blister had grown into a large gaping sore that he hadn't even felt. The next day his doctor admitted him to the hospital. The blood sugar test taken in the doctor's office was 430 mg/dl—the first clue Robert had that he had diabetes. Two days later it looked as if he might need an amputation. It took two operations and four weeks in the hospital to save his foot.

Complications of the Feet and Legs

How did a blister turn into a huge sore and almost lead to an amputation? That's what can happen when a painless sore gets infected. In someone who has had high blood sugar for some time, as Robert did (though he didn't know it), nerves get damaged. Sometimes affected feet tingle or ache. Often they have no sensation at all. This is not the blessing it might seem. Not feeling pain means not getting a message that something needs attention. Robert wouldn't have stood and walked around all day if that blister had hurt as it should have.

Robert also had partially clogged arteries from cholesterol and other fats in his blood, so the body's infection fighters couldn't get to the injured tissues in the amounts needed.

High blood sugar provides a more favorable environment for infectious organisms to grow. In addition, white blood cells don't function as well when blood sugar is high so they don't fight infections as effectively.

This combination of lack of sensation combined with poor circulation and decreased ability to fight infectious organisms is especially tough on feet.

While he recovered, Robert was given all the usual instruction about diabetes with special emphasis on foot care and a low-sugar, low-fat, low-cholesterol diet. Fortunately, he rarely drank alcohol, so he didn't need to be counseled about how alcohol aggravates nerve damage. The foot care precautions he learned included never going barefoot, preventing or quickly treating athlete's foot, inspecting feet every day for sores that might not be signaled by pain, not soaking feet, and not risking injury with "bathroom surgery."

Robert had some changes to make. He was about thirty pounds overweight, his cholesterol was 265 instead of under 200, his triglycerides (another blood fat) were 450 instead of less than 200, and, of course, his blood sugar before he came into the hospital was high. But Robert left the hospital with a good understanding of diabetes management and his new diet, a blood glucose meter, and the motivation to never let a blister turn into a medical emergency again.

Robert's complications are among those that people with diabetes worry about. We'll also discuss the tasks that are part of good diabetes care and preventing complications, why those tasks aren't easy, and some of the feelings that are associated with diabetes. You'll read about what to do and what to avoid to help your relative, friend, or co-worker with diabetes to succeed.

Causes

Many diabetes complications, including Robert's, are due to some change in the blood vessels in the body caused by the disease. Since all cells rely on the blood vessels to bring them oxygen and food and remove waste products, any narrowing or damage that causes these transportation lines to work poorly means the cells they serve suffer and may die.

Kidney and Eye Disease

Danny was a patient on the diabetes floor at a hospital where I worked. He was twenty-two years old and had had diabetes for 13 years. He'd been admitted to the hospital because of an infection that raised his blood sugar dangerously high. One of the reasons the infection had gotten out of hand is that he couldn't test his blood sugar because he'd recently lost his remaining sight. His eye doctor wanted to continue with laser treatments on his eyes but for Danny, laser therapy had only worked for a while and he'd had enough disappointment with it. He felt continuing was useless. While he was in the hospital he learned how to use a blood glucose meter with a speaker for the visually impaired.

Danny had been living alone until three months before, but his recent worsening sight had made that impossible, so he moved back with his parents. He was on the waiting list for rehabilitation classes at the Institute for the Blind which he hoped would enable him to live independently again one day.

The next time I saw Danny he was back in the hospital, groggy and sicker than ever. There was a note in his chart about drug and alcohol abuse, and he smoked a pack a day. But whatever the cause of his getting sick this time, Danny's kidneys were failing, and he was started on dialysis. He felt so bad that he didn't want to eat and he lost weight despite his nurses' best efforts to entice him with his favorite foods.

Danny probably suffered a stroke that affected his brain because he never completely regained his former alertness. Eventually he was transferred to a nursing home. Three times a week he was taken back to the hospital in a wheelchair for kidney dialysis.

We all felt terrible for Danny and his family, and we wished we could have done something to prevent the terrible consequences of his unmanaged diabetes. Diabetes educators and physicians frequently think that if they say just the right words they will provide the critical seed of motivation. Danny made some bad decisions when he was a rebellious teenager. Major complications in someone as young as Danny almost always happen after years of being in very poor control. Certainly his smoking, a major contributor to strokes and kidney failure, didn't help.

Not everyone with diabetes gets complications, though. More than two hundred people have been awarded the Quarter Century Victory Medal. To earn this medal, the recipient must have lived over twenty-five years with diabetes and be completely free of complications. Many others live decades with only minor complications. It probably helps to have good genes in addition to carefully managing one's diabetes. Since no one can choose ancestors (gene donors), a person with diabetes must rely on good management to prevent complications. And good management requires lots of motivation and hard work.

Complications of the Eyes

The blood vessels that supply cells in the eye are very tiny. When blood has a lot of sugar, it becomes thick and flows with difficulty. When thick blood is combined with high blood pressure (another frequent condition in diabetes), the tiny vessels in the eyes can bulge until they rupture. When that happens, the body tries to fix them by mending the break with scar tissue and by growing new blood vessels to supply the areas the ruptured vessels served. If no more thick, gooey blood were forced through the damaged vessels and the fragile new ones, and if the blood pressure could be reduced, there probably would be no more damage. But if high blood sugar and high blood pressure aren't corrected, more vessels will be damaged and more new ones formed. The scar tissue that is supposed to mend, may instead grow under the retina of the eye and detach it from the back of the eye. Where this happens, there is a blank spot in the person's visual field.

Laser treatments can often be successful in fastening the retina back into place. The same instrument can be used to seal off bleeding vessels.

If bleeding into the usually clear eyeball has been so great as to obstruct sight, the blood can be suctioned out, and the liquid in the eyeball can be replaced with a clear substance that allows vision.

These treatments have saved sight for thousands of people with diabetes. To be most effective, they must be started when damage is not too severe. That's why the American Diabetes Association recommends yearly eye examinations by an eye doctor who dilates the pupil with drops to examine the eye thoroughly.

In addition to yearly eye exams, the sources of the damage—high blood sugar and high blood pressure—must be controlled. This may require weight loss, a low-fat/low-salt diet, exercise, and perhaps medication to lower the elevated blood pressure. Getting the blood sugar controlled means increased vigilance with respect to carbohydrate food intake, appropriate exercise, plus testing blood and making adjustments in food and medication when indicated. This is why Danny's eye damage continued to progress; his blood sugar was too high too much of the time. He also smoked, which further constricted the blood vessels all over his body, including those in his eyes.

The leaky blood vessels and detached retina described above are parts of a condition called retinopathy.[1] It is one of the major causes of blindness in the United States, but it isn't the only eye condition brought on or worsened by diabetes.

Glaucoma is twice as common in the diabetic population and can result in reduced peripheral vision or even blindness. A gradual blockage of the normal outflow of fluid in the eye increases pressure enough to damage the neurons in the optic nerve. If diagnosed early it can usually be effectively treated with eye drops, laser therapy, or surgery.

Lastly, a cloudy lens in the eye, called a cataract, is also more common in people with diabetes. Fortunately, a cataract is easily removed surgically and a plastic lens can be implanted that restores clear vision.

---

[1] The word ending "-pathy" means "disease of" or "suffering from". Retinopathy is disease of the retina.

Kidney disease

The causes of kidney disease (nephropathy) are very similar to the causes of retinopathy. Thick, sugary blood being forced under high pressure through delicate kidney blood vessels causes damage to the kidney.

The job of the kidney is to remove waste products from the blood as it flows through the kidney. If the blood is forced through at higher than normal pressure, it causes stretching in the kidney's blood vessels. Stretching causes collagen (a fibrous substance), to form a support network that eventually thickens the kidney walls. The result is a stiff kidney that filters poorly.

Treatment of kidney disease involves controlling high blood sugar and high blood pressure. In addition, a low-protein diet can help ease the blood vessel constriction that causes higher pressure inside the kidney. If protein in the diet is reduced at the first sign of kidney damage, along with the other two treatments, damage can frequently be slowed, and perhaps the kidneys can continue to function adequately for the rest of the person's life.

Kidney damage doesn't have early symptoms that enable a person to know what's going on, so microalbumin urine tests[2] that measure tiny amounts of protein in the urine, or a blood test for kidney function, should be ordered by the doctor at least once a year. This is another reason why physician visits are so important—to discover problems like kidney damage early enough for the low protein diet, control of blood pressure and blood sugar to do some good.

If the kidneys do lose their ability to filter enough waste products and get them out in urine, they build up in the blood, making the person feel very ill. The waste products then need to be removed by filtering the blood through a process called dialysis. The most common type of dialysis is done by inserting a needle into a large blood vessel in the arm and connecting it by a long tube to an artificial kidney machine. Blood is allowed to circulate through the machine for about three hours while nurses keep a check on the patient and the machine.

A second method of dialysis, called continuous ambulatory peritoneal dialysis (CAPD), uses the peritoneal cavity in the abdomen as a filter and collection place. It involves implanting a tube called a catheter in the abdomen through which a solution flows from a bag into the body. The solution sits in the abdominal cavity for several hours attracting the waste products that are usually removed from the blood by the kidneys

---

[2] A test for tiny (micro) amounts of a protein (albumin) that is not usually present in urine. In diabetes, it may be an early sign of the kidneys' inability to save albumin for re-use by the body.

and passed out of the body in the urine. In peritoneal dialysis, these waste products pass from the blood through the blood vessel walls inside the abdomen and collect in the dialysis fluid.

Every few hours, the fluid is allowed to drain out of the body back into the bag. This process is repeated several times with bags of new fluid, until the person's blood is cleansed of many of the waste products the kidneys can no longer remove.

Some people are able to do this kind of dialysis at home themselves or with the help of a family member. They can even go shopping or travel while doing their dialysis. Judy Curtis, in her book *Living with Diabetes Complications*, tells how her dialysis was so routine that she could do it in the car, at work, in airports, on trains, and even on an airliner.

Neither method of dialysis is pleasant. Being hooked to an artificial kidney machine usually means going to a kidney center three times a week and lying on a recliner for three hours at a time. Because people whose kidneys don't work make little or no urine, any liquid they've had since their last dialysis treatment has accumulated inside their bodies. When three days of fluid is removed in three hours it leaves people feeling exhausted; their body chemistry has been altered suddenly and their blood pressure is usually low. They must also adhere to a strict diet without most fresh fruits or vegetables, dairy products, meat, beans, nuts, or salt, and very little coffee, water or other liquid— anything harmful to the body when it accumulates for days must be reduced or eliminated.

Although peritoneal dialysis doesn't require the restrictive diet since the removal of waste products is done daily, it has its own drawbacks, including chance of an abdominal infection and backaches from walking around with all that fluid inside the abdomen while the treatment is going on.[3]

After years of dialysis, whether with an artificial kidney or peritoneal dialysis, many people opt for a kidney transplant. The five-year success rate is now around eighty percent if the kidney is from a closely matched living relative. But even a kidney from an unrelated donor (usually a cadaver) has a seventy percent success rate.

Since dialysis costs around $30,000 a year, the onetime transplant expense of about $35,000 with a 70 to 80 percent chance of success is considered cost effective so it is reimbursed by Medicare and insurance companies.

---

[3] Another type of peritonial dialysis called continuous cycling peritoneal dialysis (CCPD) uses an automated machine which is programmed to exchange the dialysis fluid at periodic intervals during the night. CCPD makes it unnecessary to carry fluid around during the day, or to stop daytime activities to change bags.

The drawback to kidney transplants is that recipients must take drugs for the rest of their lives to prevent their immune system from rejecting the kidney. Anti-rejection medicines make one more prone to infections, osteoporosis, and ulcers, and they raise blood sugar! These drugs are also very expensive (about $6,000 a year), though Medicare pays for them the first three years. After that, the patient or insurance company must pick up the cost. Despite all these negatives, life is definitely more normal with a donor kidney than on dialysis.

Complications of the Heart and Circulatory System

The same fatty deposits that shut off some of Robert's blood supply in his feet might have blocked an artery supplying some part of his heart. If that had happened, Robert could have had a heart attack. If an artery in his head had been blocked, he would have had a stroke. High blood pressure adds more strain to damaged, hardened blood vessels and makes a heart attack or stroke even more likely.

Heart disease and stroke are probably the least recognized complications of diabetes, and yet if you visit a cardiac care floor at a hospital and ask how many patients have diabetes, you'd be amazed. They often go together.

Impotence

Getting and keeping an erection and normal ejaculation depend on the penis getting a good blood supply and having properly functioning nerves. Both circulation and nerves can be damaged by diabetes. Some diabetic men find it impossible to get an erection. Others are able to get an erection but have problems ejaculating.

Fortunately, there are options to remedy or at least manage male sexual dysfunction. The first is to try getting blood sugar and blood fat levels as close to normal as possible. There are also mechanical, vacuum devices that can restore the ability to produce and maintain an erection. A surgical implant is another possibility. Penile implants are expensive, but over 80 percent of the men who get them report that they are satisfied.

I remember reading a letter in an advice column in which an impotent man wrote that his doctor had offered him the option of an implant. His wife did not share his enthusiasm, however. Her response was, "I'd rather have a new dining room set."

That brings me to the last option: counseling. Just because a man has a physical reason that affects his sexual performance doesn't mean he can't also be wracked with anxiety and have that anxiety worsen the situation. Relearning sexual skills and rediscovering intimacy with his wife could enrich them both, even if none of the other options works or is acceptable to them.

Other Complications

There are dozens of other complications, varying from the mild to the severe that are associated with diabetes. Most have nerve damage, clogged blood vessels, high blood pressure, or all three in common. Some lead to damaged joints; others result in stomach and intestinal problems. Women can have problem pregnancies.

Despite the variety, prevention boils down to just a few guidelines. The same cautions and treatments are mentioned again and again. Here they are in a nutshell:

> Keep blood sugar in the normal range.
> Eat a low-fat (especially low-saturated-fat) diet.
> Limit foods with cholesterol.
> Maintain a sensible weight.
> Don't smoke.
> Don't drink alcohol without a meal or have more than 1
> drink even with a meal.
> Have yearly eye exams.
> Have yearly lab tests for kidney function.
> Exercise regularly.
> Practice good foot care.
> Have high blood pressure treated.

Preventing Complications Is Not Easy

When we hear about the serious complications that can happen to people with diabetes, we tend to think, "If I had diabetes and I could go blind if I didn't take care of it, I would stay on my diet and do everything the doctor told me."

Part of your certainty that you would do everything may be due to an unrealistic idea of just what doing everything involves.[4]

---

[4] For a detailed description of what diabetes care involves, see Chapter 5, "So Many Chores, So Little Time."

Here a is list of the daily tasks of a *perfect* patient who has Type I diabetes:

1. Test blood sugar 4 to 8 times a day.
2. Inject insulin 3 or more times a day.
3. Record all blood sugar results and times.
4. Record all insulin dosage and times.
5. Record any unusual events, such as increased exercise or feeling ill.
6. Eat meals at scheduled times.
7. Follow a prescribed meal plan.
8. Avoid concentrated sweets.
9. Limit protein in diet.
10. Eat low-fat and low-cholesterol foods.
11. Follow a weight loss or weight maintenance diet.
12. Exercise seven times a week.
13. Test blood sugar before, during, and after exercise.
14. Inspect feet daily and apply lotion.
15. Carry glucose tablets or candy and other snacks.
16. Carry meter and/or other supplies to work, school, and social events

Above are just the daily tasks. Less frequent but also essential chores include the following:

1. See doctor in charge of diabetes care two to four times a year if no problems, otherwise more frequently.
2. See eye doctor at least once a year.
3. See podiatrist every three months if feet need special care for corns, callouses, thick nails, etc.
4. Test for ketones when ill or when blood sugar is over 240.
5. Consult with dietitian if diet needs changing.
6. Buy supplies.
7. Fill out insurance forms.
8. Attend lectures and support groups and read diabetes magazines to stay current and motivated.

You might have two reactions to those lists. Maybe you said, "Wow, I had no idea what was involved in diabetes self- management. I'll be more considerate and understanding now that I know." If this was your response, give yourself a pat on the back and read on for more details.

If you thought, "That really doesn't look so bad. Some of those things only take a few minutes," you're partly right too.

Time

The time needed for specific diabetes chores may or may not seem to be a lot. It depends largely on how the person with diabetes sees the list and what is already part of his or her lifestyle. For example, for a fifty-year-old lawyer who doesn't exercise and who comes home tired every night at 7:30, being told that he must find an hour for exercise can seem a huge burden. He may say to himself, "What's the use, I don't have the time or energy, so why try?"

But for a person who never gave up exercise or who got back into the habit before being told exercise is an important part of diabetes treatment, it's like being told to keep breathing. "Noooo problem." When I ask an already accustomed exerciser how long he spends on his diabetes management every day, he's likely to say fifteen to thirty minutes.

At first I used to be alarmed by this. I'd think, "This person is not taking care of himself. He couldn't do everything he's supposed to do in less than half an hour." But he could, if he's only counting checking his blood sugar, taking insulin, recording both, and checking his feet after his shower. Those things are do-able in fifteen to thirty minutes.

And the "eating correctly" part needn't take any longer either. Or, more correctly, it doesn't take longer when it's part of an established routine. It's time consuming when a diet sheet has to be referred to or the exchange book consulted, or a person is writing out a week of menus for a dietitian to check. While someone is learning the diet and new diabetes management, it can seem as if it's taking over every waking hour. If you remember back to when you were first learning to drive, you'll be able to relate. Didn't it seem that there were fifteen things you were supposed to do simultaneously? Your instructor barked, "Watch the rearview mirror, signal a turn, don't follow too closely, slow down, take your foot off the gas, and parallel park over there." You never thought you would be able to do it all without being nervous and stressed every minute. If you've been driving for years, though, you know how automatic most of your moves have become.

That new-driver feeling comes back when diabetes is new or insulin has just been started, or a new meal plan is prescribed. The person feels swamped with pamphlets, cautions, and instructions from the physician, nurse, or dietitian (or all three), and diabetes may again seem to require constant attention to details and to the clock.

People with diabetes give a range of from 10 minutes to 2 hours per day for their diabetes chores. From discussions with them in greater depth, I know that this reflects only in part how complicated their diabetes routine is. It is more likely an indication of what they're omitting because they consider it a normal chore (exercise and fixing a meal) versus what they label as a strictly diabetes chore.

Caroline puts it this way, "I only spend about a total of 10 minutes a day, but I always must be aware of my blood sugar and how I feel 24 hours a day."

It's somewhat like going about your day while you try to remember the items you need to buy at the market later on. It means being aware of mealtimes and insulin or medication times and feelings of tiredness, nervousness, or hunger that might mean a low blood sugar reaction.

Time is not the only thing people with diabetes need. These tasks involve motivation, planning, money, inconvenience, and/or discomfort. Some, like pricking a finger to get a blood sugar level, involve more than one. Let's look at blood sugar testing, which, with injecting insulin, is either in first or second place of the most dreaded daily chore on everyone's list.

It Requires Planning and Record Keeping

Testing blood sugar requires having a supply of lancets (finger-pricking devices) and blood glucose strips, calibrating the blood glucose meter that reads the strips, and carrying strips, meter, lancets, and a log book and pen to record the results.

Insulin and oral medications must also be integrated into one's day and recorded in the log book.

It's Expensive

Buying the supplies is no small sacrifice for many people. Blood glucose test strips alone cost 60 to 70 cents each. For a person who tests four times a day, that's about $17 a week or around $70 a month. Some insurance companies pay a part or all of this expense; others do not. From my own informal surveys, people have told me their basic supplies and diabetes medicine run from $12 to over $200 a month. (Note, that this does not include any doctor fees, hospital bills, or lab tests).

It's Inconvenient and Awkward

Since blood sugar testing is most often done before meals, sometimes it needs to be done in a restaurant. Some people test in their cars before going inside. Others lay out all their paraphernalia on the restaurant table, stab their finger, put the drop on the strip, and so forth–maybe while everyone else in the party is ordering. Some go to the rest room and hope there's more than a sink ledge to perch their equipment on. It depends on the restaurant and the group of diners and how comfortable onlookers are with the procedure.

Finding a clean, private nook for taking an insulin injection can also be a challenge. (That's probably why some brave souls, experimented and discovered that they could inject *through* their clothing!)

It Hurts

Blood sugar tests generally hurt more than injections because there are more nerve endings in finger tips than in most injection sites. Sometimes the pain is over in a minute. Sometimes the finger is tender for hours. And when your friend or relative has twenty-eight or more little punctures in her fingers at the end of every week, she doesn't feel much like doing the testing that makes the pricking necessary. But she does it anyway.

It's Something *They* Say I Have to Do

Doctors, diabetes educators, mothers, and others order people with diabetes to do blood sugar testing four, six, or more times a day. Worse, they are not always understanding about any gaps in testing or undesirable results. One fifty-three year old woman says her mother still grills her about her blood sugar. If it's high, she's accused of having eaten candy; if she denies it, she's called a liar.

Blood sugar seems to be the last unrespected area of privacy to many people with diabetes.

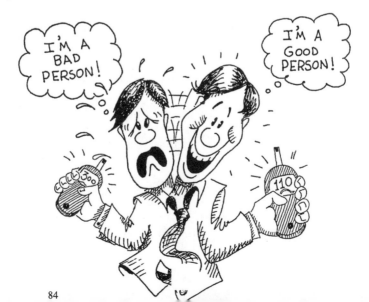

It's Frustrating

Imagine having stayed on your diet, exercised as you were supposed to, and taken your medicine on time but when you checked your blood sugar it was double or triple the normal level. For some, that happens often. One young woman told me that testing her blood sugar was like getting graded—with the chance of failing at every test. Add to that the mistaken idea of parents and others that blood sugar is perfectly controllable with diet and medicine, and you have two good reasons for frustration. It can't be controlled perfectly but everybody without diabetes thinks it can. This frustration, together with people's judgmental attitude, makes infrequent testing and made-up numbers very tempting.

The mind set that views blood sugar readings not as results that are high, low, or normal but as grades or moral judgments, makes blood sugar testing less likely to be done. The blood sugar level then becomes "bad" or "good," and by extension, the person whose blood gave that result is "bad" or "good."

If everyone considered blood sugar testing as merely a tool instead of an approval or a condemnation from on high, feeling bad could be replaced by decision making.

If I Know What My Blood Sugar Is, I'll Have to Do Something About It

Doctors tell people with diabetes to check their blood sugar regularly so they'll know when it's high or low. But lots of times your friends with diabetes don't want to know. If they know, they'll have to do something about it. That something may be injecting an extra dose of insulin, eating when they're not hungry, not eating when they are, not running with the team because their blood sugar is too high, or delaying the tennis game because they have to eat a snack first. At the very least, the blood sugar level will have to go into their log book and could bring criticism and a lecture on improving blood sugar control at their next visit to the doctor.

What Makes People Do Almost Everything They Should

You now know why diabetes management is difficult. So what keeps your friend or family member with diabetes doing any of these expensive, frustrating, time-consuming chores? People with diabetes I've talked with and who have answered my questionnaires, say that what usually keeps them on their diabetes program is, indeed, fear of complications. They may not do everything perfectly and consistently, though. The fear of a bad outcome just isn't enough to *always* overcome all the other demands on their time and resources.

Most people think it's the seriousness of the consequence that motivates someone to diligently follow a treatment. That may very well follow with a surely fatal disease like, some kinds of cancer. After the patient is convinced of the operation's necessity and agrees to have it, he has the operation, he goes for chemotherapy or radiation treatments, and eventually he's done with the whole thing. With diabetes there's never an end to the treatment, and it's the patient that does almost all the work, not the surgical team or the technicians in radiology. Diabetes requires lifelong day-in and day-out discomfort, expense, food sacrifices, and inconvenience. Motivation needs to be found again and again.

No matter how serious that possible outcome is, most of the time it is the number and difficulty of the tasks and adaptations that determine whether the person will follow the diabetes management plan or not.

Think of health routines you may or may not be following. If you're a woman, you probably go to the doctor for a yearly pap smear. But do you do a monthly self-exam of your breasts? If not, is it because you're not sure it's necessary? Or maybe you're not sure you know how to do it perfectly. Or you need to sign up for a class to learn how but you don't have transportation, or it costs $15 and you're short this month. Or perhaps your doctor doesn't ask you if you do it and reward you with a "good work" when you say you have, so you think it can't be so important, after all. In short, it's very easy for a physician to say, "You need to do this, it's important." But you know that the doing is much more complicated.

Another example is flossing your teeth. Do you do it every day? It's hard to remember to make that part of your bedtime or after-meal routine, isn't it? If it is a habit, you don't need to remember—it's automatic.

Diabetes management is like that. It's hard to make all those tasks habits, but once they are, they become second nature. That's one of the reasons this book stresses helping the person with diabetes to stay on track and not break good habits. It can be hard to get them back again once temptation has been tasted. Try to put yourself in the shoes of someone with diabetes: imagine a time when you made a list of New Year's resolutions. You were going to lose weight, quit smoking, or practice piano regularly, or something else that probably would be good for you. How many of those resolutions did you keep? For how long? Yes, it's tough changing old habits even when the goal is a worthy one.

Fortunately, other motivating factors can come into play when the burden of changing routine is great or the fear of complications seems less compelling. My patients mention not wanting to feel tired or sick, the challenge of seeing how well they can do, accepting diabetes as something they just have to deal with, and wanting to be alive with loved ones. But these attitudes usually come with some experience and maturity.

Parents have an especially hard time instilling the motivation to eat sensibly, test, and take insulin on time into their teenagers. What seems to work best with this group is to emphasize how taking care of themselves can help them be and stay independent. Discussing goals and how good control can help realize these goals is also useful. No one can play well in sports or realize a dream of being a good *anything* if high or low blood sugars are sapping energy.

You can't do it for your child. You can provide the tools and offer help with working through problems without giving unsolicited advice. You can help your teenager see and understand himself or herself. But discovering the benefits of taking good care of oneself is a one-person job.

How Not to Help

> Don't say, "You should" or "You shouldn't."
> Don't say, "You never" or "You always. . ."
> Don't say, "You can't" or "You must . . ."
> Don't judge.
> Don't nag.
> Don't criticize.

When you do any of these things, you are coming from a place of superiority. You think you know what's wrong and how it should be solved. However, unless you have a chronic disease that requires the work that diabetes requires, admit that you don't *really* know what it's like. And even if you're right about what's wrong and how to solve the problem, the person may do the opposite rather than let you be proved correct.

Imagine the feelings of the fifty-three year old woman whose mother accused her of eating candy whenever her blood sugar was high. Even if it were true, could she correct the problem without admitting that her mother was right? Would she *want* to prove her mother right? She'd be giving her mother proof that nagging works!

How much more effective it would have been if her mother had said, "I see your blood sugar is above the range you're trying to stay in. Is there anything I can do to help?" This shows respect for the other person's feelings and a willingness to work this out *with* the person instead of having him or her *do it alone.*

Keep the long-term picture in mind. Don't become the enemy in order to be right once or to hear the doctor side with you.

Now let's look on the positive side and see what you *can* do to help.

How You Can Help

1.   *Describe, don't judge.* In the above example, the helper described the blood sugar as "above the range" but did not evaluate it as a "bad" blood sugar due to some dietary indiscretion. Or if she had noticed that her daughter had had cake that afternoon and maybe that was why her blood sugar was up, she could say (if it's true), "I notice that you've been eating sweets this week. Do you feel under more stress than usual?"

2.   *Be specific.* In the example above, the mother pinned down the behavior to this week. It makes it clear than there is some recent change that may have a specific cause, not just the person's "badness" or "laziness."

3.   *Show empathy.* Imagine that your friend or family member has just told you about the time his or her diabetes was diagnosed. This is usually a milestone in a person's life, on a par with the birth of a baby–it changes one's whole life. An example of a pitying remark would be, "You poor thing." This makes the person think you see him or her as a helpless victim. A better, more empathetic response would be, "I had no idea that you went through all that." You could open up further understanding by asking, "Is having diabetes as difficult as you imagined it would be when your doctor gave you the diagnosis?"

4.   *Welcome positive changes.* This sounds as if it doesn't need mentioning. Of course you would applaud health-promoting changes. Not necessarily from the bottom of your heart, though. You might see time at the gym as time stolen from you and the family. Or a support group

could seem threatening because those people understand having diabetes in a way you never could. That understanding might mean bonding in a way you think you can't compete with.

Sometimes you can join the gym, too, or accompany your special someone to the support groups and learn. Or, if that's not possible, it would be best to accept and adjust. It is important, though, to recognize the resentment for the natural thing it is and grow from the experience.

5. *Help keep temptation away.* This could be as simple as not having foods high in fat and sugar around the house or office. It can mean choosing restaurants with healthy choices, or preparing low fat meals with fresh fruit for dessert. It could mean educating friends who put your family member or friend in situations where they are less likely to take care of themselves (like going out to drink every night after work).

When I ask diabetics, in general, what they wish friends, colleagues, and family members would do make it easier to control their diabetes, they say, "Don't have stuff I can't eat around." At one diabetes educator's meeting, when I asked that question three dietitians simultaneously said, "Don't bring Oreos in the house." (At 47 calories and 2 grams of fat each, Oreos may not seem *so* bad but dietitians know that nobody stops at one). Many diabetics say they feel bad when people eat sweets in front of them. If we care about someone, we don't want to be the cause of their sadness, do we?

How much of a sacrifice would it be to not have unhealthy food available? (After all, there are many other opportunities to eat junk.) I've known a severe asthmatic whose husband and son would go outdoors to smoke. I was also a guest at a Thanksgiving dinner where wine and spiked egg nog weren't offered because one of the invited relatives was a recovering alcoholic.

You read how Pat's husband helped her by allowing her to banish the donuts. Pat tried to carry this a step further for other people. She helps out at a church where men's groups have meetings. The standard refreshments are huge platters of cookies. Pat suggested that maybe they could offer fruit instead of, or at least in addition to the cookies. She was hooted down by the refreshment committee. But, she hasn't stopped trying. And I hope she doesn't. "Most of the those men are overweight and could use a little less temptation," Pat added.

Rome wasn't built in a day, Pat's husband didn't sprout wings and a halo overnight, and maybe your family or group will need a little persistent bargaining.

For that social or office group, maybe just the *addition* of a healthy snack (like the fruit platter Pat suggested) will at least give some options to folks whose diet plan doesn't include cookies.

The next time your church, temple, or other group suggests an event with refreshments, how about suggesting a baking contest or pot luck with only low fat and/or low sugar foods?

Try expending a little extra effort in making the low-fat, low-sugar treat look terrific. Fruit kind of takes care of itself with its great colors but other foods like fat-free muffins may need a cherry on top or decorative paper liners. Bring out the paper doilies, tiered cookie plates, and novelty cookie jars.

Another reason for keeping junk food out of sight is to reduce "pay backs." Pay backs happen when people deny themselves treats but later "reimburse" themselves.

For Martha it worked like this: yesterday she passed up the donuts at the office, the pie in the company cafeteria, the chocolates a colleague passed around the office, and the dessert on the pastry tray at dinner (and she really *loves* eclairs). At home, as she was cleaning up the living room, she found a half-full bag of chocolate chip cookies her son had left on the sofa. She had denied herself four times that day. "That amount of sacrifice deserves a reward," she told herself, and down the hatch went five cookies. And she didn't even feel the guilt that splurging usually brings, because, from her point of view, she'd "earned" those cookies.

It needn't have happened, though. If Martha had had fewer temptations that required will-power to overcome, she might never have had her "cookie-compensation" event. If you are a friend, fellow worker, husband, or son of someone like Martha, you can be a great help in keeping the total of her tempting moments to a minimum, thereby lessening "pay back."

Part of keeping temptation away is to help the person with diabetes not feel different. It's hard to have to choose between being like everyone else and "being good." If no choice needs to be made, staying on one's diabetes management plan is easier.

6. *Be patient.* This refers to the times you have to wait for your friend to have a snack before you can start your bike ride, or times you have to eat earlier than you'd like because of his or her schedule. It includes trotting off to get some juice when a low blood sugar hits. The more irritation you show, the guiltier your friend, co-worker or family member will feel and the worse you'll feel when you reflect on your impatience and lack of understanding. Again, recognize and accept your

resentment as natural, but work on doing better next time. There's got to be at least one inconvenient trait you have that is irritating at times.

7.   *Set a good example.* If you were considering losing weight, or switching to a low-fat, low-cholesterol diet, starting to exercise regularly, or quitting smoking, do it now and be a good example. You may be able to commiserate and praise each other. When one of you is ready to jump off the wagon, one can save the other. The roles will be reversed from time to time when weak moments come.

Being a good sport and joining in should pay off in a healthier you and a healthier someone with diabetes.

8.   *Praise.* Finally, people with diabetes say praise from you, the people that are important to them, is a positive force. Make it sincere and recognize a positive effort or result. A "Good work on taking your blood sugar after dinner," or "I saw that you exercised almost every day this week" is the kind of pat on the back that is likely to motivate the person you're applauding to test after dinner or to again exercise frequently in the future.

Chapter 8
Low Blood Sugar: When Sugar Is Medicine

There is one situation where your knowing what to do in a hurry might be vital. That's when someone with diabetes has low blood sugar, also called an insulin reaction, insulin shock, or hypoglycemia.

What It Feels Like To Jo

"My mouth gets dry and my tongue feels thick. *Rivers* of perspiration run from my scalp and forehead. I get shaky and rubber legged, somewhat disoriented, but 'something' kicks in and I'll grab one or two glucose tabs or glucose gel. When I first got diabetes, I followed the dietitian's orders and drank orange juice or ate three graham cracker squares. The problem with those orders was getting my hands to take orders from my brain, so sometimes the orange juice didn't make it to the quivering glass. After the juice, I would *try* to wait twenty minutes for results (as the dietitian also told me to do), but the symptoms always got so much worse before they'd start to get better. I'd find myself tearing into a candy bar to speed things up. Now I just start with glucose or hard candy. This works better for me.

"In public or when someone is at home with me, I sometimes suddenly begin talking a blue streak, stuttering and jumpy. My husband knows what this means, and he'll ask me if I could be 'sliding.' In my insanity, I get very provoked and will go into a snit or even pout. This isn't *me*. Towards the end of the second piece of the candy treatment, I'll understand what's going on and can at least express my appreciation for his efforts.

"When I get low blood sugar in a grocery store or church, I feel profound dread and embarrassment. There I am, fumbling with candy wrappers while people look at me suspiciously.

"At night I sometimes wake up freezing cold and soaking wet, having no idea of where I am. Instinct kicks in, I search for "warm," so my husband becomes alerted and starts squirting glucose gel into my mouth while I'm giving him a hard time. I try to get away from him and the stuff he's trying to put in my mouth. My brain is so vacant, I'm sure that he's the one with the problem, not me. Once he manages to break into that fog (he'll holler or shake me, get me to sit up if he can), I'll very grudgingly cooperate.

"After Bill, or I (if I'm alone during the day) get past the worst by eating the candy, I know I have to eat something more substantial to keep my blood sugar up, but the all-over sick feeling doesn't lend itself to appetite. I eat anyway.

"I feel wiped out physically, as though I've climbed Everest. I'm weak as a kitten and can barely lift my arms, walk, or sit upright. This can persist for hours.

"At night I may fall back to sleep, but I don't rest and wake up feeling truly awful."

The Morning After

Jo's experience of feeling achy and unrested in the morning is shared by many diabetics. Even when they haven't awakened and been fed candy or glucose, their blood sugar in the morning may read in the 400s (normal is 80[1] to 120 mg/dl). That's because their own emergency blood sugar raisers have treated the low blood sugar—a little too late to prevent the low blood sugar symptoms and a lot more than ideal or the reading wouldn't be 400. It can take half the day to bring this high a blood sugar back into the normal range.

Wondering Why It Happened

Jo's husband lovingly "grills" her about what could have caused her low blood sugar. Did she eat all of her bedtime snack, did she take too much insulin, did she remember to compensate for her exercise in the afternoon? Even when there's no one else that asks piercing questions, the diabetic asks them and feels guilty. He or she "must" have done something wrong to have caused this. Feeling guilty is not helpful. Asking questions to try to prevent a future low blood sugar caused by similar conditions *is* useful.

---

[1] 80-120mg/dl is considered the ideal blood sugar level. However, first thing in the morning 70-110 is normal and after a meal, up to 180 is acceptable.

You as a helper need to remember that although most low (and high) blood sugar episodes can be prevented by good diabetes management, not all of them can. A perfect blood sugar is not possible without a cooperative pancreas.

What Could Cause a Low Blood Sugar

From the questions that Jo's husband asked her when probing for the cause of her latest low blood sugar, you can see that the usual ones have to do with food, insulin (or oral medication), and exercise. Specifically, a meal that's too small, has too little carbohydrate, that's late, or worse, skipped, is a frequent cause of low blood sugar. For people who take insulin or oral blood sugar-lowering medication, food has to be eaten when the medicine is at its peak of action.

A very bad idea is to take insulin and then get behind the wheel to drive to a restaurant. Driving under the influence of insulin (or blood sugar-lowering pills) when the last meal's food is long gone is dangerous. Lots of things could happen that would delay getting to the restaurant or getting served that could be at least embarrassing, at worst, tragic.

Another cause of low blood sugar is too much insulin. That could be because too much was drawn up in the syringe. Or it could have been injected into a thigh or other part that got exercised shortly afterward, so the insulin was absorbed more quickly than expected. Sometimes insulin needs are reduced because the person has lost some weight or has reduced food intake to try to get in better control, or has started exercising regularly which can improve his body's response to insulin.

Too much exercise is the last of the trio. Actually, it's not *excessive* exercise that causes the low blood sugar, but the fact that the exercise wasn't compensated for by either reducing the insulin (before or afterwards), or increasing food (before, during, or afterwards). Diabetes and strenuous exercise are not incompatible, but like so many things about diabetes, even normal activities have to be planned.[2]

Robert Polhill, an insulin-requiring diabetic, who was held hostage in Lebanon for 39 months had about 400 low blood sugar reactions during that time. Many of his low blood sugar reactions happened because his captors would insist he perform some unscheduled exercise like cleaning the room. The only treatment provided for low blood sugar was to drink some of the cola the guards provided for that purpose.

Twice he didn't feel the low blood sugar soon enough and passed out. The other hostages managed to drizzle enough cola down his throat to

---

[2] Exercise is discussed later in Chapter 13.

bring him out of shock. This was extremely risky since he could have inhaled the cola while he was unconscious, but in this situation, there was no other option. Thank goodness it worked.

The three most common causes of low blood sugar, then, are too little food, too much insulin, or too much exercise. There is a fourth cause, however: alcohol. Alcohol is such an important issue for the diabetic that it deserves a section of its own.

Alcohol and Low Blood Sugar

When a person with diabetes drinks alcohol the blood sugar can become too low. This is because when anyone—diabetics and nondiabetics alike—drink alcohol, the liver stops doing one of its most important jobs, which is to release stored sugar when needed. Whenever we go several hours without food, our liver supplies us with sugar to tide us over until we eat. But when we drink alcohol, the liver only processes the alcohol and stops doing other tasks.

So alcohol, without food to keep the blood sugar up, is potentially dangerous for someone with diabetes. A single glass of wine with dinner is not dangerous, however, because the food in the meal will supply enough sugar to keep the blood sugar from getting too low, so the reserve supply in the liver will not be needed. The point is that alcohol can be safely consumed in moderation (one or, at most, two drinks), but only with a meal.

> These have equivalent amounts of alcohol:
> 4 ounces wine
> 12 ounces beer
> 1 ½ ounces liquor

Another serious safety issue is that it's difficult for the person with diabetes and for his or her friends to tell when the person is tipsy or experiencing low blood sugar. Symptoms of low blood sugar include confusion, poor coordination, and slurred speech. Is this person drunk? Would you know whether to put this person to bed or to treat him or her for low blood sugar? Probably not. And the person with diabetes would be too confused to tell you.

This is why moderation is not a word used lightly when drinking and diabetes are discussed. For example, in the case of a person with slurred speech, or any other symptom shared by both low blood sugar and alcohol excess, I would try to get some juice and/or food into him or her and have someone spend the night checking the person every half hour for excessive sweating, tremors, or coma in case the blood sugar gets dangerously low.

Early Symptoms of Low Blood Sugar

The early symptoms of low blood sugar are the same ones (though less severe and shorter) you may have felt when you were afraid or angry. They occur when adrenaline is pumped into the blood stream to prepare you for "fight or flight." It's a reaction to something your body thinks is an emergency. And since the body perceives low blood sugar as an emergency, it feels and looks very much like extreme fear or rage. The symptoms are:

> Hunger
> Sweatiness
> Shakiness
> Nervousness
> Irritability
> Light-headedness
> Headache

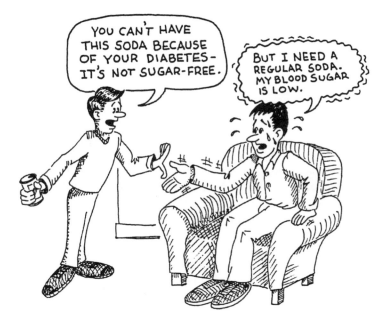

Treatment

If the symptoms are caused by low blood sugar, eating something with sugar is the "cure." Surprised? Maybe you thought people with diabetes are allergic to sugar and always have to avoid it. Not so. A low blood sugar is an emergency situation that must be corrected, and sugar does the job.

If the diabetic is aware of the symptoms, he or she will probably reach into a pocket for glucose tablets, or get a regular soft drink or some juice. Now is *not* the time for the usual sugar-free soda—the person needs sugar and needs it quickly! One of the following treatments for low blood sugar is recommended:

> ½ cup fruit juice or nondiet soda
> 1 tablespoon honey
> 1 tablespoon sugar
> 4 - 6 Lifesavers
> 2 - 3 Glucose Tablets (check package-other brands have smaller tablets, give enough to equal 10-15 grams carbohydrate)
> ⅓ - ½ tube Insta-Glucose gel (1 tube has 30 grams carbohydrate)

What works quickest is glucose tablets or gel (glucose starts working in two minutes). Next speediest is sugary liquid such as non-diet soda or fruit juice. It only takes ½ cup (4 ounces) to do the job. This is not a case in which "if a little is good a lot is better." *The goal is to correct the low blood sugar and bring it back to normal, not to shoot it past normal into the high range.*

A low blood sugar reaction is also not the best time for a candy bar. A chocolate bar is about 50 percent fat. That fat actually slows down the sugar which needs to get from the digestive system into the blood. So give glucose tablets or gel, if available. If not, some hard candy such as Lifesavers work well.

Years ago the treatment for low blood sugar was a *big* glass of orange juice with a spoonful or two of sugar stirred in. That must have kept blood sugar from dropping again for a very long time. It also shot it through the roof. In those days, however, you couldn't test someone's blood just anytime, so no one knew what that twelve-ounce glass of juice did to the blood sugar. Now we know better.

Back to your role as helper in this low blood sugar event: with the early symptoms listed above, your only job will be to fetch and carry if the person with diabetes asks for your help. But if the low blood sugar goes untreated until it gets much lower, a whole new set of physical signs can appear and you may need to do more.

The human body is a wonderful organism with many emergency backup systems. For example, there is one hormone (insulin) that lowers blood sugar. But there are several that raise it. That's because a blood sugar that is so low that it results in starved brain cells is such a catastrophe that the body has several ways to combat it.

The first warning is the set of symptoms that are early signs of a low blood sugar: the sweating, nervousness, and so forth. They are indications that adrenaline is working to make the liver release its emergency supply of stored sugar. Unfortunately, there's not an inexhaustible supply, especially in people trying to maintain near-normal blood sugar, so sometimes you, the helper, must do some or all of the correcting.

Symptoms of More Advanced Low Blood Sugar

Later symptoms of low blood sugar are due to brain cells being starved for glucose. They include the following:

> Confusion
> Lack of coordination
> Slurred speech

The person with these symptoms urgently needs your help. The confusion alone may prevent the diabetic from knowing what he or she needs to do. *You* must know and take steps.

Treatment for Moderately Advanced Low Blood Sugar

The treatment is still the same. If the person is conscious, you can give ½ cup of soda or fruit juice in small sips or offer glucose or hard candy. Any of these things is OK unless the person has passed out.

Symptoms of Advanced Low Blood Sugar

A low blood sugar that is not corrected may continue to get lower. The brain cells become starved for glucose, and they stop functioning. The symptoms of severe low blood sugar are:

> Convulsions
> Loss of consciousness
> Death

You must never pour something into an unconscious person's mouth (unless you're hostages). He or she could inhale the liquid or food and choke. It wouldn't get into the stomach, but into the lungs. If glucagon is available and you know how to use it, this would be a good time to get busy and do it.[3] If not, call 911 or get the person to an emergency room. (See *Calling for Help* later in this chapter for what to say on the phone to the dispatcher).

Using Glucagon

An injection of glucagon (pronounced "glué-ka-gon") is necessary only if the person cannot eat or drink because he or she is unconscious or having a seizure. It is rarely needed, but when it is, it is very needed.

There is nothing difficult about giving a glucagon injection. It can be given in the front of a thigh, or in the upper outer arm, or anywhere you have seen the diabetic take insulin (such as in the fat over the abdomen). You won't do any harm, and you might do a tremendous amount of good.

If you are extremely nervous about whether this will work, call for the paramedics and then give the shot. That way you know that if you don't do it just right, your backup is on the way, but you won't be letting the low blood sugar get worse.

The only tricky part of giving glucagon is mixing it up. It usually comes in a box that contains a syringe with liquid in it and a bottle with powder in it. The powder is the glucagon. It's left in a dry form so it can be stored longer. You have to add liquid to make it injectable.

The liquid in the Lilly Emergency Kit is in the syringe that comes with the powder. Take off the needle cap and inject all of the liquid into the bottle. Shake a bit to mix. Then pull back on the plunger to draw out the glucagon liquid. If the diabetic is a child, take out only half the liquid. For an adult, take it all out. Don't worry that if you give too much, you will overdose the person. Glucagon is not a medicine that needs to be precisely measured the way insulin does.

Take your thumb off the plunger, if that's where it is, hold the syringe by the barrel (the long part), and push the needle quickly into the arm (or wherever you decide to inject). Now put the thumb holding the syringe on the plunger and push in the fluid.

Occasionally someone will vomit after getting glucagon, so turn the person on his or her side so no stomach contents will get inhaled.

---

[3] Glucagon is a natural hormone produced by the pancreas that raises blood sugar. It must be injected like insulin.

Usually the person can be roused in five or ten minutes. Give sips of juice or sugar in water as soon as he or she awakens.

If you have never given a glucagon injection before, you may be scared at the thought. Jo's husband is, and he's grateful that he has never had to use it. Still, he and Jo are glad it's there, just in case.

You can rehearse for the day you might have to use the kit by walking through the steps without actually mixing or giving the glucagon. Know where the kit is. Look at the bottle and syringe. Leave the cap on the needle, pretend you are injecting the solution, and so forth. Even pretend to give the injection to your friend or family member with the needle cap still on. Or, better yet, offer to give the person an insulin injection. Many diabetics really appreciate a chance to have a shot in a place they can't reach easily, and you will have a chance to get over the scariest part at a time when the "injectee" is able to give instructions. You will feel much better about the real thing after any trial run.

Interestingly, although you don't need a prescription to buy insulin, you do to buy glucagon. If your family member or friend takes insulin and does not have a glucagon kit for every place he or she spends a lot of time, encourage the person to ask the doctor for a prescription. It will just take a phone call to the doctor and a phone call to the pharmacy.

The best place to store glucagon is in the refrigerator. It doesn't really need to be kept that cold (anything under 90° F. is safe) until it's mixed, but it's an easy place to find it). You probably will never need to use the glucagon, so it will eventually expire. If there is a kit around the house or your diabetic colleague's office, ask to see the expiration date. It may need replacing. If it does, you can use the expired kit to practice actually mixing up the solution before you throw it all away. Be sure to dispose of the needle as is mandated in your state. Some states require only that you break off the needle and put it in a crush-proof container; others want the needle and syringe placed in a specially marked disposal box and taken to a medical waste dump. Nowadays in this age of AIDS, custodians and garbage collectors get understandably upset when they get stuck with a hypodermic needle.

How Common Is Serious Low Blood Sugar?

Clearly, low blood sugar is not to be taken lightly. The good news, however, is that low blood sugar events that require help are not everyday events (except for people with unusual conditions like Jo).[4]

---

[4] Jo has frequent low blood sugar because her pancreas was removed due to severe pancreatitis. Without a pancreas, she has no beta cells to make insulin and no alpha cells to make glucagon. On top of that, because of her surgery, she can't accurately predict when her food will leave her stomach and start entering her blood stream, so it's hard to get her food and insulin in sync.

Recent studies have reported that as few as 4 percent and at most 25 percent of insulin-treated people have one or more episodes of low blood sugar a year that require the help of someone else.

Irritability and Low Blood Sugar

The symptom most family members think they can recognize as a sign of low blood sugar is irritability.

At the first hint of testiness, they will say things like, "Don't you think you better have some juice? Your blood sugar must be low." This almost universally makes people with diabetes angry. (I used to be puzzled by this because I figured if I were in that situation, I would rather someone think I was having a low blood sugar than think that I was a grouch). But this is not how people with diabetes see this. Here are some of their comments:

> "Ask me what is bothering me to determine if
> I'm really upset or if a low blood sugar is
> controlling my emotions."

> "Leave me alone unless I'm showing obvious
> symptoms and am not in control of what I'm doing."

> "Just remember everyone has a bad day now and
> then. Don't assume it's from diabetes."

Another reason for not jumping to the conclusion that irritability is due to low blood sugar is that irritability can mean just the opposite. The following is a common complaint:

> "Learn the symptoms of both high and low blood
> sugar and know how to deal with each, as needed.
> I get crabby when my blood sugar is *high*."

People with diabetes have all the emotions other people have. Sometimes they have something to be irritated about.

It wouldn't be a good idea to insist that someone have juice if they didn't need it. You would raise a normal or high blood sugar higher and incidentally, might make the person crabbier.

Also, the same symptoms that alert you to a possible low blood sugar could be the result of some other emergency. Even if you eliminate anger and fear, a heart attack or shock could be to blame. Keeping an open mind could mean catching a serious condition in an early stage.

What To Do When

If the person:	Do this:
Is irritable	Ask what is wrong.
Is shaky or sweaty	Offer to bring soda (*not sugar-free*), juice, or candy.
Is confused, uncoordinated, or has slurred speech	Give ½ cup soda, juice, glucose, or other sugar.
Is unconscious and you know how to inject glucagon	Prepare glucagon, inject, and turn on side in case of vomiting. Give soda or juice when conscious.
Is unconscious and you cannot inject glucagon	Call paramedics or take person to an emergency room.
Is unconscious, you can't inject glucagon, and there's no phone or transportation near	Put glucose gel, honey, or syrup between gums and cheeks and stroke to encourage swallowing. (Some authorities are afraid that even thick substances can get in an airway, but if no other option is available you need to do *some thing*).

How to Be Sure It's a Low Blood Sugar

Fortunately, you no longer need to guess whether blood sugar is low or high if you know how to take a blood glucose reading with glucose strips and, preferably, a meter. Below 60 is considered a low blood sugar and should be corrected. A blood sugar of 60 to 70 could need correcting soon—test again in fifteen minutes. A reading of 70 to 120 is in the safe, normal range.

If you can't check the blood sugar level, the safest rule is that if the person cannot get his or her own juice or sugar because of confusion or lack of coordination, you should assume it's a low blood sugar and treat it. That's because a low blood sugar can become an emergency in minutes, whereas a high blood sugar usually takes several hours, or even days, to become serious.

Calling for Help

In this time of scarce medical resources, it's very important to be as efficient and accurate as possible when you deal with the call screener at the emergency dispatch switchboard.

The person you talk to first has to understand or be convinced that what you're reporting is a real emergency. He or she will probably pull it out of you eventually—but you can effectively cut to the chase and speed your friend's treatment by saying something like:

"My close friend (or whatever your relationship is) has lost consciousness, has diabetes, and is very likely suffering a low blood sugar emergency."

After the Low Blood Sugar Is Corrected

Glucose and sugar work quickly, and that's why we use them to raise low blood sugar. However, they also wear off quickly—in about thirty minutes. The person recovering from low blood sugar will need something more substantial to keep the blood sugar from falling again.

A good snack would be:

½ peanut butter or cheese sandwich
and
1 glass skim milk

Or if the next meal is due soon, don't wait—serve it now.

A low blood sugar doesn't have to be frightening. Just know how your friend or family member's behavior changes when his or her blood sugar is out of control and do what is indicated.

Diabetics tell me that their friends and family generally do the right thing when they have low blood sugar. Only about 30 percent say someone *once* should have done something differently and not one said he or she was put in danger because of a mistake.

Helpers Sometimes Do Too Much

The most common mistake in low blood sugar episodes is for helpers to overreact. Some relatives yell and blame. Other people tend to panic. Untrained friends and colleagues are prone to call an ambulance even when the person is conscious and says he or she is really all right and is recovering.

One Swedish exchange student said his friends insisted on taking him to an emergency room despite his protests. He finally let them, just so they'd learn he was really OK. However, he wasn't used to our medical care costs in the United States. He says the shock of the $200 hospital bill for a blood test, sandwich, and a five-minute chat with a doctor came a lot closer to killing him than the low blood sugar had.

Professionals Sometimes Do Too Little

There is no guarantee that just because someone is a nurse, doctor, or paramedic, he or she will always make the best decision the first time.

Kira tells of a time when she was sixteen and was driving long after she should have had her dinner (she was trying to lose weight by skipping a meal). She passed out and smashed into a parked car. She was able to give her home phone number to a witness. Her mother wasn't home but her sister was and rushed to the scene of the accident.

The police arrived before her sister, so Kira told them, "I have diabetes, I have low blood sugar." But the police officer kept asking, "What kind of drugs are you on?" In her confusion, Kira insisted she was a werewolf, which only reinforced the officer's and the newly arrived paramedics' belief that she was on drugs. Her sister came during all this, pointed to Kira's Medic Alert bracelet, and asked for glucose, but all they wanted to know was, "What kind of drugs is she on?"

Kira was then taken to an emergency room, where the staff refused to give her anything to eat or drink because they needed to check her blood for drugs. Meanwhile her blood sugar was getting lower and lower. Finally Kira's mother arrived, yelled at a nurse, and at last succeeded in getting her some juice.

These professionals all forgot the first rule of helping a confused or unconscious person you know has diabetes. *When in doubt, treat the person for a low blood sugar.* It will do little harm to give glucose tablets or juice if the person can swallow, or a shot of glucagon, if he or she can't. And if there's no improvement, other causes for the condition can *then* be considered.

The moral of this story is that you can do much better than that police officer, those paramedics, or that emergency room staff. You can check for a medical I.D. bracelet, insist that top priority be given to what it says, and you can yell like that mom for juice or get it yourself.

Chapter 9

High Blood Sugar

Martha's flu started with a headache, fever, and muscle aches. The next day she felt worse, called in sick, and stayed at home. She tested her blood sugar (it was a little high, but not alarmingly so), took her usual morning insulin, fixed herself a bowl of canned soup, and spent the morning sipping a two-liter bottle of sugar-free soda.

In the afternoon Martha felt worse and went to bed for a nap. When she awoke, it was dark. She hadn't eaten lunch and her stomach was upset, so she didn't want even soup. She was afraid that if she took her evening insulin without eating, her blood sugar would get too low, so she just took another bottle of sugar-free soda to the bedroom and went back to bed. She didn't check her blood sugar because she wasn't eating anything, so how could it be high? And anyway, she was just too tired.

Martha had to get up twice at night to urinate, which was unusual for her, but she figured that with all the soda she was drinking, that was to be expected.

The next morning Martha felt truly awful. She felt nauseated, her mouth was dry, and she was barely able to drag herself to the bathroom for what seemed the hundredth time. She did take her blood sugar, though, because she wasn't sure if she needed to take insulin or not since she couldn't bear the thought of eating. Her blood sugar was 486![1] Martha called her doctor. Her doctor did not tell her to take two aspirins and go to bed. He told her she needed to get to the hospital right away, and if she didn't have anyone who could drive her, he'd call an ambulance! Martha called her sister, who got her to the hospital within an hour.

When Martha got to the emergency room, a nurse took her blood sugar. This time it was 502, Martha was breathing rapidly, she felt and looked flushed, and her tongue and lips felt as parched as a desert. A urine test showed ketones, and a blood test showed that her blood had become acidic. Diagnosis: ketoacidosis.

Martha was so dehydrated that she needed fluids by vein to replace what she'd lost in all those trips to the bathroom. She also needed salts and minerals. What she needed most of all was insulin. Ketoacidosis is caused by a severe shortage of insulin.

---

[1] Normal blood sugar is between 70 mg/dl and 110 mg/dl first thing in the morning and under 180 mg/dl after meals.

Martha spent a day in intensive care getting intravenous fluids with salts and minerals added to replace what she'd lost. Her blood sugar was taken hourly, and all her urine was tested for ketones.

Her sister spent the day in the waiting room worrying.

The next day Martha was better and could be transferred to a bed on the regular diabetes floor. Her doctor had the nurse diabetes educator give Martha a refresher course on what to do anytime she's sick. Martha had a lot of questions for the nurse. Here are Martha's questions and the nurse's answers:

Why did my blood sugar get high even though I wasn't eating anything?
Sugar doesn't come just from food you eat. It can come either from the liver's stored glucose or from new sugar the liver can make from protein. So even though you knew you weren't taking in any sugar in food, you were getting a hefty supply from your liver.

Why did my liver "think" I needed more sugar?
Your body was fighting off a flu infection and needed extra energy to handle the stress of your illness. Your liver will do the same thing with any major stress like surgery, a heart attack, or a stroke. Emotional stress, even good news, can raise blood sugar. One young woman never had a high blood sugar with ketones until the day she found out she was finally pregnant.

Even if you hadn't been sick but needed extra energy, a low insulin level would have signaled the liver that it needed to give up some of its stored glucose. That's one of the ways the body tries to keep an even blood sugar between meals.

I guess I shouldn't have stopped taking my insulin then, right?
Right. You still needed insulin to get sugar into the cells, but none was available. When the sugar started accumulating in your blood, your kidneys tried to flush it out.

But I drank lots of fluids as you're supposed to when you're sick.
Yes, you did. That was good strategy, and it might have been enough for someone who didn't have a shortage of insulin and high blood sugar.

I know I'm in the hospital for ketoacidosis and not just dehydration. Why did I get ketoacidosis?
When your cells couldn't get enough sugar to function, the body tried to

supply an alternate fuel supply—it used stored fat. The trouble with fat is that it releases by-products that produce toxic ketones and make the blood acidic. Neither of these is healthy. You felt nauseated and started breathing more quickly, all as a result of burning fat. Your body needed insulin, fluids, and food to function well.

But I felt sick to my stomach. I tried soup, but when I got sicker I don't think I could have kept any food down.
Soup was a good idea. Another food that seems to be tolerable when a person feels nauseated is saltine crackers. Ask any woman who ever had morning sickness what she was able to keep down, and you'll soon have a list of foods for sick days.

If even soup and crackers are out, you still need some calories, especially some carbohydrates to balance the insulin. Fifteen grams every one to two hours is recommended. Here is a list of some foods that have 15 grams of carbohydrate:

$^1/_2$ cup Jello (not sugar-free)	$^1/_2$ cup apple juice
5 Lifesaver candies	$^1/_2$ cup orange juice
6 saltine crackers	3 glucose tablets
8 animal crackers	1 cup Gatorade
3 graham crackers	1 cup milk
1 slice toast	$^1/_2$ cup ice cream
$^1/_2$ cup cereal	$^1/_2$ cup fruit yogurt
$^1/_2$ cup pop (not sugar-free)	tea with 3 teaspoons sugar

If you can't drink a glass of juice all at once, sip it slowly so that you get $^1/_2$ cup down every hour. Some people find a regular Popsicle (again, not sugar-free) refreshing, and it melts so slowly that even an upset stomach can handle it.

It doesn't sound as if $^1/_2$ cup of fluid an hour is enough when you're sick.
You're absolutely right. It isn't enough. You still need to drink at least 1 cup (8 ounces) an hour of sugar-free liquid to keep you hydrated.

Is that all I need to do, eat, drink, and take my insulin?
No, you need to check your blood sugar at least four times a day when you're sick. If it's over 240, test your urine for ketones.[2] If the test shows

---

[2] Strips for testing ketones can be bought without a prescription at a drug store. Foil-wrapped strips keep about 2 years before they expire.

even slightly positive two separate times, call your doctor. Even if you don't have ketones, if your blood sugar is over 240 at two different times, call your doctor.

It's possible that the doctor can keep you out of the hospital by suggesting an adjustment in insulin, if it's done early enough.

Another thing the doctor can do is prescribe something to counteract the nausea so you can keep eating and drinking enough to stay out of trouble.

This sounds like a lot of work for someone who feels terrible and just wants to sleep.
It is, and that's why it would be best if you weren't alone when you're sick. It's very helpful to have someone bring you fluids, remind you to check you blood sugar or do it for you, and call the doctor if you get worse or don't improve in 24 hours.

Ketoacidosis can be deadly if not treated early enough.

What kinds of things should my helper call my doctor about?
You or your helper should call if you:

Have vomiting, diarrhea, or stomach pain.
Have not been able to take fluids and keep them down for four hours.
Have a fever over 100° F.
Have a blood glucose level over 240 twice.[2]
Have ketones in urine twice.
Have breath with a fruity, sweetish, or acetone odor.

Martha went home the next day with a pamphlet on sick day management. Her sister made her promise to call her or *someone* the next time she was sick. She said giving Martha soup and Jello was better than wringing her hands in a hospital waiting room any day!

Who Usually Gets Ketoacidosis?

There are three common situations when ketoacidosis occurs. The first is in people who don't know they have diabetes. The second is when insulin is not taken, and third is when an infection or other illness causes the liver to release stored sugar.

---

[2] There may not be ketones in the urine of someone with very high blood sugar if they have Type II diabetes. They can still become very dehydrated and develop a potentially fatal condition called hyperosmotic coma.

1. People Who Don't Know They Have Diabetes

Ketoacidosis is rare in someone who produces insulin, so the people most at risk are those with Type I diabetes. About a quarter of people newly diagnosed with Type I diabetes have ketoacidosis. When John was diagnosed, he did not have ketoacidosis.[3] He had frequent urination, thirst, hunger, and weight loss, which are all symptoms of high blood sugar. He had some ketones in his urine (ketonuria), but he had not yet gotten to the point of ketoacidosis.

Kira[4] did have ketoacidosis by the time she was diagnosed. She had all the symptoms John had, plus vomiting and dehydration.

Sarah, who was sixty-five years old when she was diagnosed, had a mild case of ketoacidosis, although her diabetes turned out to be Type II. She had been so thirsty because of her not-yet-discovered diabetes that in the days before she was hospitalized, she drank quarts of juice. The vast amounts of sugar in all that juice, combined with her already insufficient insulin production, caused her to produce ketones.

Sarah recovered so quickly that her doctor planned to discontinue her insulin when she was well enough to leave the hospital.

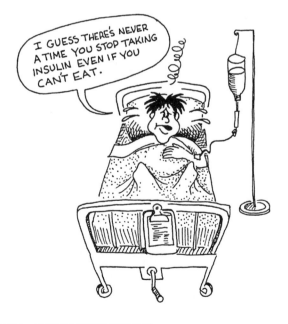

---

[3] The story of John's diagnosis is in Chapter 3.
[4] Kira's story is in Chapter 15 on diabetes and kids.

2. People Who Reduce Or Omit Their Insulin Dose

Reducing or omitting an insulin dose is the most frequent preventable cause of ketoacidosis.

Sometimes the reasons seem sensible, as they did for Martha, but it's just not a good idea to guess and assume that insulin should be stopped. The doctor should be in on the decision and it should be based on blood sugar readings.

3. People With Infections

Respiratory, urinary, and intestinal infections are the most common infections. Martha had a respiratory infection, which was enough to raise her blood sugar and start the whole cycle of ketoacidosis and dehydration.

Next September, when the influenza vaccine again becomes available, Martha should get a vaccination, thereby reducing her chances of getting the flu by 80 percent. The flu vaccine is recommended for everyone with diabetes over six months of age. It is considered safe for pregnant women, a lot safer than getting the flu during pregnancy, which could harm mother and fetus.

Even those with kidney disease or heart or lung disease should be vaccinated. The downside is a sore arm. Martha will tell you that beats tubes in your veins in the intensive care unit.

Pneumonia vaccine is also recommended for folks with diabetes. It only needs to be taken every 10 years, or so.

Why Ketoacidosis Gets Out of Hand

The symptoms of ketoacidosis are frequently ignored because they could be due to a dozen different conditions. Flu frequently causes an upset stomach, so people like Martha don't think of ketoacidosis. Some even get a tender and swollen abdomen, which suggests gas or an inflamed appendix or other problems instead of ketoacidosis.

Finally, low blood sugar is so tiring and scary that people with diabetes work hard to prevent it. They learn that insulin must be balanced with food, so when they can't eat, they think omitting their insulin is a good idea. They forget that food is not the only source of sugar and that the liver can supply sugar too.

What If Ketoacidosis Doesn't Get Treated in Time?

Martha was lucky that she called her doctor while she still could. She might have gotten so weak and sick that she could have gone to sleep and never awakened again. That sleep could have changed into a diabetic coma. She might still have gotten treatment in time to be saved, but only if someone had found her before she became one of the 3 to 10 percent who die of irreversible coma or one of the other fatal conditions caused by dehydration and related problems.

How You Can Help

Nurses consider themselves "the patient's advocate." You, too, can be an advocate by looking out for your friend or family member's best interest when they're sick. Call at least once a day, and visit if you can. Heat soup, help with blood sugar testing, or do whatever he or she will let you do.

You may by able to prevent someone with diabetes from jumping to the wrong conclusion (for example, thinking that their vomiting is merely from eating a bad piece of fish), or from taking their illness too lightly and not testing often enough or not calling the doctor.

It's important, if you do visit, to take a good look at the person. Look for rapid breathing, a flushed face, drowsiness, and slow reflexes. This could mean ketoacidosis. At the least, it means it's time to call the doctor.

Chapter 10
The Diabetes Diet: More Than Just No Sugar

Why do some people with diabetes carry snacks?
Why do some diabetics avoid only sugar while others also limit fat or
    protein or all three?
What's the exchange list you've heard some of them follow?
What kinds of desserts can diabetics eat?

If you share time with someone with diabetes, chances are you've wondered about some of these questions. This chapter gives you the answers and the basic information to understand the answers. It tells you
what diabetics need to learn about food to follow a diabetic diet and how
they and their dietitians or physicians adapt such a diet to the diabetic's
preferences and medical needs.

You'll probably be surprised at how little difference there is in the
foods that are good for you and the foods that are good for the person
with diabetes.

Sugar Has Its Place

Many folks believe that people with diabetes are allergic to sugar, that
they should never eat it, and some even think that eating too much sugar
is what caused diabetes in the first place. But eating too much sugar
doesn't cause diabetes, and sugar doesn't have to be avoided completely.
In fact, it can't be avoided completely because almost everything we eat
is, at least partly, turned into sugar in our bodies. And, as discussed in
Chapter 8, sugar is taken deliberately in a concentrated form to normalize a blood sugar that is too low.

What Foods Turn Into Sugar

Our cells need food in the form of a particular sugar called glucose and
our body changes foods of all different kinds into that sugar. Not all
foods change completely into sugar, though. About 90 percent of carbohydrate foods like bread and cereal become glucose, about 30 percent to
60 percent of protein foods like egg whites are converted to glucose, (although the process is slower than the metabolism of carbohydrates), and
less than 10 percent of fat becomes glucose. Since carbohydrates change
almost completely and fairly quickly into sugar, the more carbohydrate

a food contains, the more it will contribute to raising blood sugar soon after it's eaten.

You may think, then, that carbohydrate foods should be avoided, and that only proteins and fats should be eaten. And, in fact, avoiding carbohydrates was the only treatment for diabetes before the discovery of insulin. That kind of diet prolonged life for people with no other options. But with today's treatments, it's neither necessary nor desirable for diabetics to eat only eggs, meat, and certain vegetables such as cabbage and celery.

Carbohydrates Are Necessary

Our bodies need carbohydrates for fuel, and provided they're eaten in the right amounts at the right times, they're essential nutrients even for people with diabetes. In fact, about 50 percent of our calories should come from starchy foods like cereal, rice, and bread.

Protein Is Not The Perfect Food

Protein is needed to build and repair tissues, but it has been so overemphasized that many people eat more than enough, sometimes at the expense of other nutrients that are equally important. In fact, many North Americans eat several times the amount of protein they need. When a greater proportion of North Americans were so desperately poor that they lived on corn or rice, meat and dairy products were such a rarity that they really did need more protein in their diet. Nowadays, it's more likely to be the corn and rice and other starches that need boosting.

But more serious than eating too much meat and dairy products and not enough of something else, is the strain that eating a lot of protein puts on the kidneys. People who have had diabetes for more than fifteen years may begin to show kidney damage caused by years of high blood sugar and high blood pressure. Cutting back on protein for these people can slow down further damage and delay or even prevent the need for kidney dialysis or a transplant.

Too Much Fat Is Too Darn Common

Too much fat is a problem for most of us, but it is compounded for people with diabetes because of their greater risk for clogged blood vessels, which can result in strokes, gangrene, and heart attacks. Foods high in saturated fat are of special concern since they are the ones generally believed to cause clogged blood vessels by raising cholesterol in blood. Here's a list of some of the foods that are high in saturated fats and cholesterol:

beef	hot dogs	hamburgers	most cheeses
pork	sausages	eggs	whole & 2% milk
lamb	lunch meat	butter	ice cream
bacon			

Also any food that says on the label that it contains *hydrogenated* oils should be limited. That's because when vegetable oils are hydrogenated (to make margarine, for example), they become saturated fats.

Cholesterol-rich foods and saturated fat are not the only concern. Calories from *any* source that we eat beyond what we immediately need is stored in the body—much of it as fat. Since most of us in the industrialized countries are not at risk of starving, we don't need a lot of stored fat.

Fat is singled out as the food component we most need to limit partly because it is so rich in calories. It doesn't take much fat in addition to our carbohydrate and protein needs to put us over the number of calories we need and cause us to store it as flab. In addition, fat doesn't require much processing to store since it's already in the form of the final storage product—fat. Since carbohydrates and proteins use up significantly more calories in the process of changing into fat, you'd have to eat more of these to make a pound of fat.

Still, no matter what that extra stored body fat started out as, it contributes to poor blood sugar control. This is especially true of people who get diabetes in later years—they are very often overweight. That extra padding interferes with insulin's function, so more insulin than the body can produce is needed. That's the insulin resistance that is so common to Type II diabetes. The result? Sugar accumulates in the blood and blood sugar goes up. Those who can lose their extra fat can often stop taking insulin or pills.

A Body Shape That Is Especially At Risk

Where a person carries that excess fat can be as important as having extra fat to carry. The apple-shaped person is at greater risk for cardiovascular disease than the pear-shaped person. (Apple-shaped refers to those whose fat is predominantly carried above and around the waist; pear-shaped, predominantly below the waist). Those who are shaped more like an apple, have more metabolically active fat that is more easily deposited on the inside of arteries.

The pear-shaped person is less at risk for a heart attack or a stroke. It seems that the fat around the thighs and below the waist is not the same kind that is in arteries.

Not that being pear-shaped is *healthy*, it's just not as *unhealthy*.

What if you're not sure which body type you or your family member, friend, or colleague is? All you need is a tape measure to find out. Measure the waist and then measure the hips. Divide the waist measurement by the hip measurement. Here's what the numbers mean:

Less than 0.75 = pear-shaped

0.75-0.80 = mildly apple-shaped

More than 0.80 = very apple-shaped

The apple-shaped person needs to get very serious about doing whatever is necessary to lose that around-the-waist fat.

A Recommended Balance Of Carbohydrate, Protein, And Fat

No one kind of food is all bad or all good. All of us need protein, carbohydrate, and fat in our diet every day. It's the amounts of each that nutritionists find to be unhealthy in the typical American diet. Here's a comparison of our sources of calories:

Typical American Diet	Recommended diet
30% to 40% carbohydrate	50% to 60% carbohydrate
12% to 18% protein	12% to 18% protein
40% to 50% percent fat	25% to 30% fat

Notice that I said "our" calories. The above percentages are recommended for nondiabetics too. So if you eat healthily for yourself, including cutting down on sugar, salt, and fat, you won't need to prepare anything different for the person with diabetes.

The Exchange List

It would be possible for a diabetic to write a list of the foods he or she planned to eat for the day, look each up in a nutritional table, and calculate the amount of carbohydrate, fat, and protein in each food. The person could then calculate the percentage of the total calories each group had. On the first few tries, the numbers wouldn't match those in the recommended list above. So he or she would have to add some foods and subtract others. It would be a lengthy process. There must be an easier way. And there is.

The exchange system for meal planning was developed to simplify food calculations and thereby meal planning for people with diabetes. In this system, foods are grouped together in "exchange groups" with similar carbohydrate, fat, protein, and calorie amounts.

The list that organizes foods in this way is called the "exchange list," and each group is called an "exchange." The groups are called exchanges because, in the specified amounts, all the foods within each exchange group can be exchanged for each other. I'll explain what is meant by "specified amounts" shortly.

The Exchange List[1]

Carbohydrate	
Starch	**Vegetables**
bread	asparagus
cereals	broccoli
corn/peas	cabbage
crackers	carrots
pasta	onions
beans	tomatoes
potatoes	**Fruit**
rice	apples
Milk	bananas
milk	grapes
yogurt	oranges
	peaches

Meat/ Meat Substitute	Fat
meat	avocado
poultry	bacon
cheese	butter
eggs	cream
fish	cream cheese
tofu	margarine
	oil
	peanuts

---

[1] You can get the 32-page exchange list from the American Diabetes Association. Your local affiliate will mail you one. To find your local affiliate, look under "Diabetes" in your phone book.

You're probably surprised to see some of the foods in what seem to be the wrong group. Remember, though, these foods are classified as to their composition of carbohydrates, fat, and protein, not the food group classification system you learned in school. For example, although we think of peas as a vegetable, they actually have so much carbohydrate, or starch, in them that they are nutritionally closer to bread than they are to beets, bean sprouts, and broccoli. So within the carbohydrate group, starchy vegetables such as peas and corn are separated from vegetables with little carbohydrate such as broccoli and cucumbers.

Another list with surprises is the fat list. An avocado is so fatty (88 percent fat), that it is considered a fat exchange, not a vegetable. Peanuts are 76 percent fat, not at all mainly a protein food, as most people believe.

Each serving of a food in each category has a certain number of grams of carbohydrate, protein and/or fat and a certain number of calories. Before we discuss what constitutes a serving, here's what the terms *gram* and *calorie* mean:

A *gram* is a measure of weight from the metric system. There are 28.35 grams in an ounce. Three grams weigh as much as one penny, so you can see that it is a small quantity.

A *calorie* is a measure of energy. Technically, it's the amount of energy necessary to raise the temperature of one gram of water one degree Centigrade. Food energy is measured in thousands of calories, called *kilocalories* but most people, even nutritionists, speak of these units as calories.

The list below gives the number of grams of carbohydrate, protein, and fat, and the number of calories in one serving from each exchange group. A serving size may vary considerably from item to item, as we'll discuss later. What's important is that the number of grams does not change within each category.

Amount (in grams) of Nutrients in One Serving from Each Exchange List

Exchange Group	Carbohydrate grams	Protein grams	Fat grams	Calories
Carbohydrate				
Starch	15	3	trace	80
Fruit	15	0	0	60

Milk				
skim (non-fat)	12	8	trace	90
low fat	12	8	5	120
whole	12	8	8	150
Vegetable	5	2	0	25
Meat				
lean	0	7	3	55
medium-fat	0	7	5	75
high-fat	0	7	8	100
Fat	0	0	5	45

Remember, foods in the same group have different portion or serving sizes even though the number of grams of carbohydrate, protein, fat, and calories is the same. For example, a normal serving of most cold cereals is 3/4 cup. A serving of Grapenuts, however, is only 3 tablespoons, while a serving of puffed rice is 1 1/2 cups. Varying the portion sizes allows all the cereals, or whatever foods are similar, to be in the same exchange list. One cereal can be exchanged for another, but the serving size may need to be adjusted.

The exchange list suggests many other possible trade-offs. The same 3 tablespoons of Grapenuts can be exchanged for 1/2 bagel or 1 slice whole wheat toast, or a 6-inch tortilla.

Of course, as you've probably guessed, it's not always this simple. We don't always eat a food that's only carbohydrate or only protein. Even bread is a mixture of carbohydrate and protein and we eat many dishes like pizza that have ingredients from more than one exchange list. Foods like pizza are called combination foods. In diabetes nutrition guides some popular combination foods have the number of starch, fat and protein exchanges itemized so that exchanges can be figured without too much effort.

Here are some foods from the combination list:

Combination Foods

	Serving size	Exchanges per serving
Casseroles	1 cup	2 carbohydrates, 2 medium-fat meats
Cheese pizza (thin crust)	1/4 of 10"	2 carbohydrates, 2 medium-fat meats, 1 fat
Vegetable beef soup	1 cup	1 carbohydrate
Pot pie	1 cup	2 carbohydrates, 2 medium-fat meats, 4 fats

Calculating a Diabetic Diet

When Anthony, a sixty-two year old overweight office manager, was told he had Type II diabetes and needed to follow a diet, he expected to be handed a printed sheet with some menus on it. That's what had happened to a friend of his. Anthony was afraid he wouldn't do any better than his friend did on the printed diet—it had almost nothing on it his friend liked and was so boring that he ate more that *wasn't* on the diet sheet than *was*. A couple of weeks of that diet, and his friend had higher blood sugars than before he tried it.

Fortunately for Anthony, his doctor sent him to a registered dietitian (RD). This is someone who has completed college and postgraduate training in nutrition and has passed a national qualifying exam. The dietitian made a meal plan that took into consideration Anthony's nutrition needs, how physically active he is, his schedule, and his food preferences, plus his doctor's recommendations (lose weight, no insulin or oral diabetes medication until diet and exercise have a chance to work).

The Interview with the Dietitian

The dietitian first asked Anthony's height, which was 6'1". From his height, plus his age, body build (medium), and sedentary lifestyle, the dietitian calculated a sensible weight for him (185 pounds) and from that reasoned that a 1,500-calorie diet would be a good starting point. That may seem like a very small number for a man who is 6'1", but Anthony had a sedentary job and needed to lose weight. When he reached his goal weight of 185 he would be able to add up to 700 calories to his daily total. If he added exercise, he could either add some calories right away or tough it out and get down to his goal weight more quickly.

The dietitian then used 1,500 calories to calculate how many calories of carbohydrate, protein, and fat Anthony should eat every day. She then translated calories into grams and, finally, into exchanges.

At this point the dietitian got creative. She asked Anthony a number of questions about his meals. Did he like milk? If so, was he willing to switch from whole milk to nonfat milk? (He was). Did he feel meat at lunch and dinner were musts? (Yes, he certainly did). Was bread and butter a staple for him at every meal? (No). Did he usually have a snack before bedtime? (Yes).

Based on Anthony's answers, the dietitian allocated the grams of each nutrient. She tried to spread them fairly evenly so that he got some carbohydrate, protein, and fat at each meal. She also tailored the exchanges to match his preferences. For example, he said he wanted meat for lunch and dinner. Even lean meat has some fat, and since Anthony had only 50 grams of fat for the whole day, some careful choosing had to be done. She left out some of the cheese, margarine, and whole milk she might have included for other clients but included enough fat and protein exchanges at lunch and dinner so that Anthony could pick a lean meat from the exchange list.

Personal Preferences are Important

Anthony's dietitian considers her clients' personal preferences and schedules very important to her client's achieving their desired goals. She always inquires about her clients' likes and dislikes for milk, eggs, meat, and other foods because most needs can be accommodated by making choices that still supply the desired amount of protein, carbohydrate, and fat.

For example, some people hate skim milk and would rather have bread without margarine or a bagel without cream cheese than give up their 2 percent fat milk. Others want their red meat (even if it is only a little 3-ounce piece) rather than twice as much shrimp. And people who want their glass of wine with dinner may find giving up two fat exchanges a small price to pay for their 4 ounces of Chardonnay.[2]

A meal plan should reflect a person's taste or it probably won't be followed.

What the dietitian came up with for Anthony was the following daily total of exchanges:

Carbohydrate exchanges	15
Meat exchanges	5
Fat exchanges	7

The dietitian then distributed the various exchanges among three main meals and a bedtime snack.

The Role of Snacks

Snacks can serve several purposes. In Anthony's case a bedtime snack was written into his meal plan because of his personal preference. If he had been taking insulin or oral medication, it might have been essential to keep his blood sugar from going too low in the middle of the night.

---

[2] A 3-ounce glass of Chardonnay has 100 calories.

For people who like to eat frequently (sometimes called "grazers"), the dietitian might plan between-meal snacks to prevent hunger pangs that could lead a desperate grazer to go off the meal plan.

People on insulin or pills frequently have mid-morning and mid-afternoon snacks if they need to match their medication's peak effect with some food. Frequently, three meals a day are not sufficient to balance the peak action times of insulin or oral medicine. To prevent a low blood sugar due to medication, the dietitian may reserve some food exchanges from meals for one or two snacks. *These snacks are not treats to be added or left out on a whim.* They prevent insulin or pills from lowering blood sugar too much between meals.

It might sound nice to have someone "order" you to have a snack but it's not much fun to have to stop what you're doing to eat, not because you're hungry, but to accommodate an insulin or oral medication effect. An understanding physician will try to adapt the medication schedule to the person's meal and daily activities, not the meals to the insulin, but it's not possible to avoid some disruptions.

Eating on a Schedule

Insulin or no insulin, scheduling mealtimes can be somewhat flexible. While it's not possible to safely skip a meal when one is on insulin or pills, a plan can usually be designed with a wide array of meal sizes and times. Everything from a small early breakfast, to a big late lunch to a light supper, to no snacks, to three snacks, or almost any combination you can think of, can usually be accommodated.

For people who work unusual hours, such as evening or night shifts, meals can be divided to adapt to this pattern, but long periods without food should be avoided. What can't be done easily is to change the agreed upon meal plan schedule on a moment's notice.

This is one of the main gripes people with diabetes have. And this necessity for eating on time is not just irksome for the person with diabetes. It causes countless problem situations with friends and family members, and sometimes colleagues and managers at work, who don't understand that eating on time is not just a personal quirk or a bid for control, but a medical necessity.

Learning to Use the Exchange Lists

There are three parts to a diabetic eating plan:

1. Timing
2. Portion sizes
3. Type of food

Timing

Often the dietitian works with the physician to balance meal times with the action times of insulin. Even with Anthony, who is not on any diabetes medication, timing is of concern to the dietitian. Not because he could have a low blood sugar reaction if he didn't eat on time, but because Anthony needs to space meals fairly evenly to avoid feeling so hungry that he'll go overboard when he finally does eat. Not only would he probably eat many more calories, but his blood sugar would probably rise to a level that he couldn't bring back to normal for several hours. To prevent this, the dietitian spreads the exchanges out fairly evenly and urges Anthony not to delay meals more than an hour, and not to skip meals.

Portion Sizes

For people like Anthony who are on no medication and are overweight, restricting calories is the main consideration. To make sure he doesn't overdo on calories, Anthony needs to learn what portion sizes are compatible with weight loss and what kinds of food have the most nutritional value with the least calories. So part of the dietitians's job is to teach Anthony what a sensible piece of meat looks like (one meat exchange is one ounce, so the usual three-exchange meat portion is only the size of a deck of cards). Most of us are not accustomed to thinking of that as a serving. Restaurants and butcher shops have trained us to expect BIG, THICK slabs as normal. To educate Anthony, the dietitian showed him plastic models of food servings. She also urged him to weigh his food for awhile to learn what appropriate amounts look like.

Type of Food

In addition to portion sizes, Anthony's dietitian explained the disadvantages of eating foods high in fat (especially saturated fat) and cholesterol. Diabetics are prone to have high cholesterol and other blood fats (triglycerides are one example). Anthony's blood test revealed that his total cholesterol level was 250 mg/100 ml. Of that 250, his "good" HDL cholesterol was only 30, while his "bad" LDL cholesterol was 220.

Another way of assessing the risk in good versus bad cholesterol, is to divide the total cholesterol result by the HDL cholesterol value. In Anthony's case, if we divide 250 by 30, we get 8.33. Ideally, the ratio of total cholesterol to HDL cholesterol should be less than 4.5. If Anthony can raise his HDL to 40 and lower his total cholesterol to 180, he will have reached that healthier ratio.

Here are Anthony's blood fat levels and the normal levels that would lessen his risk for a heart attack and stroke:

	Anthony's Blood Fats	Normal Blood Fats
	mg/100ml	mg/100 ml
Triglycerides	415	60-220
HDL cholesterol	30	Over 40
LDL cholesterol	220	Under 130
Total cholesterol	250	Under 240[3]

Anthony's results mean that he is at moderate risk for a heart attack or stroke. The risk comes from the accumulation of cholesterol deposits on the inner walls of blood vessels; these deposits damage the vessel walls and reduce blood flow.

Cholesterol is carried through the blood by proteins called lipoproteins. "Good" high-density lipoproteins (HDL) remove cholesterol from blood vessels and protect against heart disease.

"Bad" low-density lipoproteins (LDL) carry cholesterol from the liver, where it is made, to the blood, where it may get deposited if there is not enough HDL to remove it. (One way to remember which is which is that in school a *high* grade is *good* and a *low* grade is *bad*).

It may seem from this explanation that cholesterol is just a trouble-maker, but the liver produces it for some very good reasons. Cholesterol is an important component of bile acids (important for digestion), sex hormones, vitamin D, and hormones of the adrenal gland, such as cortisone.

Useful as cholesterol may be, Anthony has too much of it. He can reduce it by eating fewer cholesterol-rich foods (egg yolks, dairy products, and meat) *and* less of the raw materials the liver uses to make excess cholesterol–saturated fats. Adding soluble fiber in the form of apples, oat bran, beans, etc. can also reduce cholesterol. By exercising, he can increase the level of his good cholesterol, thereby improving the HDL/LDL ratio. If those three strategies don't work, he can take cholesterol-lowering medication.

Most saturated fats come from animal products (meat and dairy products) but margarine can be made from unsaturated vegetable oil by adding hydrogen molecules. Thus, it becomes saturated and solid at room

---

[3] This figure applies to men over forty and is fairly liberal. Some sources say anything over 200 is too high.

temperature, a characteristic of saturated fats. Exceptions are palm and coconut oil, which are saturated and liquid at room temperature.

Because Anthony was on a reduced-calorie diet, his dietitian had already cut out a lot of foods high in cholesterol and saturated fat.

She showed him the fat exchanges she included on his meal plan and explained the importance of limiting himself to seven exchanges a day. She verified that he knew what foods to avoid or to eat only in tiny amounts. They reviewed the differences between different oils.

Polyunsaturated oils (corn, safflower, and sunflower) are believed to lower cholesterol levels. Monosaturated oils (olive, canola, and peanut) may also do so but their effect is less certain. Either is preferable to saturated fats, but both have lots of calories (125 calories per tablespoon), so they should be used sparingly.

A helpful way to cut down on fat is to know how to calculate the percentage of fat in a food. Anthony's dietitian taught him how to look at a label of a packaged food and calculate the percentage of fat. This is the formula:

1. Multiply the grams of fat per serving by 9. (There are 9 calories in a gram of fat).
2. Divide that number by the number of calories.
3. Multiply this number by 100.
4. The result is the percentage of calories in that food supplied by fat.

A sensible guideline is almost always (except on one's own birthday) to limit foods to those that are under 30 percent fat. Although it's true that some foods such as bread, have little or no fat, others such as salad dressing, that are 100 percent fat, can wipe out the benefit of the bread in a hurry. That's why low fat salad dressings are such a help. Cookies and pastries are less likely to have equally delicious, commonly-served low fat versions so they are usually very high in fat. For example:

Percentage of calories from fat

Glazed doughnuts	47%
Lorna Doone shortbread cookie	45%
Bear claw Danish pastry	54%

One of the habits Anthony had that added lots of saturated fat to his diet and contributed to his weight gain, was helping himself to a Danish or two every morning at the office. His company supplies these donuts or pastries as a favor, but they're no favor to Anthony.

The dietitian explored with Anthony how best to deal with this temptation. He could ask that the pastries be stopped, thereby risking being labeled a bad guy by his co-workers. Plan number two was asking that instead of pastries, fresh fruit be provided. That too could result in unhappy office colleagues. His third option was to bring fruit or yogurt from home and eat that instead of a Danish. (Incidentally, if you have a colleague with diabetes, please back him up if he suggests healthier snacks, or propose them yourself).

Another problem for Anthony is the frequent office birthday parties and other events with cake and cookies. His dietitian suggested that he take only a sliver of cake and then stand as far away from the "temptation table" as possible.

But not everything is a no-no. The dietitian tried to show Anthony that he doesn't have to avoid everything. She encouraged him to eat lots of vegetables and whole grains for the fiber they provide—not only because fiber can lower blood sugar, but because foods with fiber tend to be more filling.

She also urged Anthony to get his fruit exchanges by eating whole fruit instead of by drinking juice. She explained that he would be able to eat a larger, more satisfying portion of whole fruit, plus get more healthy fiber for the same number of calories.

And, of course, she explained what foods contain concentrated forms of sugar and how to substitute other foods or sweeteners. (I'll say more about sugar substitutes later in this chapter and in Chapter 11, "Inviting Someone with Diabetes to Your Home for a Meal").

When Anthony left the dietitian's office with his first meal plan, that was not the end of his instruction on diet. Most dietitians ask clients to write out several menus of their preferred foods, using the exchanges allotted for each meal. The client brings this back in a few days or a week so the dietitian can verify whether the client understands the exchange system and if the number and placement of exchanges on the plan is realistic for him. For example, if Anthony complained that he felt as though he were starving at four in the afternoon, the dietitian could take a fruit exchange away from breakfast or a milk exchange from dinner to allow for a 3:00 P.M. snack. Or since Anthony could still lower his blood sugar and lose weight (although more slowly) eating 200 calories more a day, the dietitian might just add a snack or two up to that calorie limit.

That kind of "fiddling" is helpful in tailoring a meal plan to the person.

Here is a sample dinner Anthony wrote out that fits in with his 1500-calories-a-day meal plan using the exchange system:

What the Dietitian Wrote as Meal Plan	What Anthony Chose from the Lists
3 meat exchanges	*3 oz baked chicken*
5 carbohydrate exchanges	*1 cup boiled potatoes* (2 exchanges) *and 1 small dinner roll* (1 exchange) *1/2 cup carrots* (1 exchange) *and lettuce-wedge salad* (free) *1 cup fresh strawberries* (1 exchange)
1 fat exchange	*1 tablespoon French dressing* (1 exchange)
Free beverage	*black coffee with artificial sweetener*

Fortunately, there are some foods such as diet soda, coffee, bouillon, dill (not sweet) pickles, and lettuce that are considered "free foods" and which can be eaten at any time without measuring or exchanging.

The exchange system may sound cumbersome, but people who use this system get very adept at looking at a plate of food and making a good educated guess as to the number of starch or meat, etc., exchanges that are there, and what they should eat and what they should leave so they don't overshoot their meal plan.

So no fair nagging people with diabetes to clean up their plates.

Other Diabetic Diets

An exchange diet is not the only diet recommended for people with diabetes. Anthony's dietitian probably chose it because he needed to learn what was a reasonable portion size and to control his fat as well as his carbohydrate intake. The exchange diet was a useful tool for Anthony's nutrition education.

Other diabetic diets include a sugar-restricted diet, a weighed-exchange diet, a high-fiber/high-complex-carbohydrate/low fat diet, a constant-carbohydrate diet, and a low carbohydrate/high protein diet.

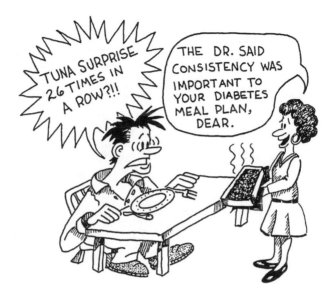

Anthony's exchange diet already urges limitation of table sugar (sugar-restricted diet) and portion size measuring and weighing (a weighed-exchange diet). The dietitian also suggested that Anthony eat substantial amounts of fiber, complex carbohydrates, and limit fat (high-fiber/high-complex-carbohydrate/low fat-diet).

The constant-carbohydrate diet is for people who take insulin. The goal is to keep the amount of carbohydrates constant at each meal and snack. If the person eats less carbohydrate, the insulin dose is reduced.

Anthony is getting four diets rolled into one. His diet also adheres to principles of good nutrition that everyone should follow:

Eat a well-balanced diet.

Restrict sugary foods.

Reduce fat, especially cholesterol and saturated fat.

Increase fiber.

Maintain a sensible weight.

Avoid excessive protein and salt.

There is also the low-carbohydrate/high-protein diet used by some insulin-dependent diabetics who have a great deal of trouble controlling their blood sugar. This diet, and others, addresses different problems from ones that Anthony and most diabetics have.

The variety of approaches to "managed eating" is just another reason why a registered dietitian is such a valuable ally in choosing and planning a meal plan.

Sugar and Sugar-free Foods

It's easy to assume that any food that says "sugar free" is OK for someone with diabetes. Wrong. Another common error is to think that "sugar-free" means there is no carbohydrate in the food. What "sugar-free" means, legally, is that the food has no table sugar (sucrose) but may have corn syrup or fructose (fruit sugar), any one of the other four sugars (galactose, lactose, maltose, and glucose), or some other sweetener that has calories and can raise blood sugar to some degree.

Another legal requirement is that the ingredient used in the largest amount by weight be listed first, the next greatest is listed next, and so on. Sometimes food companies use several different sweeteners so no one sweetener is present in sufficient quantities to require having it at or near the head of the list of ingredients. The manufacturers hope this gives consumers the false impression that the product has negligible amounts of sweeteners when the total amount might actually be quite significant.[4]

More on Diet Foods

There's probably a section in your supermarket set aside for dietetic foods which you might think would be a dandy place to find lots of food for diabetics. The first problem with foods labeled "dietetic" is that "dietetic" does not mean "diabetic." A dietetic[5] product may be for a low-salt or some other diet and not be designed for the diabetic's needs at all. Also, even if some products are made with the diabetic in mind by using artificial sweeteners instead of some type of sugar, most of them are not low-calorie. A candy bar made for diabetics has just as much fat in it as a normal candy bar. Only the sugar is missing, and by now you know that most people with diabetes need to watch their fat and calorie consumption at least as much as their sugar intake. Most dietetic products, except for diet jelly and fat-free salad dressings, are no great improvement over regular foods, despite their higher prices.

People who are insulin-dependent and who need to watch their sugar intake closely, but who don't have a weight problem can eat most sugar-substituted foods in moderation. But even they cannot make them a staple in their diet for two reasons: first, some of the artificial sweeteners, such as sorbitol, can cause diarrhea, and, second, the saturated fat in

---

[4] See Chapter 11 for more on shopping and cooking for someone with diabetes.
[5] Dietetic means "pertaining to diet." The word doesn't indicate what kind of diet it refers to.

chocolate and other dessert products can contribute to high cholesterol levels. Alas, a truly harmless diabetic dessert (except perhaps sugar-free gelatin) has not yet been invented.

Is It Sugar and Is It Bad?

Unlike coffee, tea, and diet sodas, which don't raise blood sugar, all foods and especially sugars do, to some degree. Table sugar, honey, corn syrup, maple syrup, other, so-called simple sugars or simple carbohydrates, and anything containing these used to be thought of as invariably quick raisers of blood sugar and therefore to be avoided except to treat low blood sugar.

However, new nutrition research has shown that although these sweeteners may raise blood sugar quickly when eaten alone, if they are taken in small to moderate quantities with a meal containing fat, protein, and complex carbohydrates (such as pasta), they don't necessarily cause the blood sugar to skyrocket. The trick, though, is that they must be eaten in small amounts, eaten with a meal, and something must be omitted to accommodate the exchanges in the treat.

How Desserts Can Be Part of a Sensible Diabetic Meal

In the sample dinner Anthony wrote for his dietitian, he was entitled to have five carbohydrate exchanges, two of which he met with 1 cup of boiled potatoes. Instead of the potatoes, though, he could have had a slice of angel food cake without frosting or 1/2 cup of sherbet. Because these desserts are concentrated sources of carbohydrate, the portion sizes are, unfortunately, very small. Even if Anthony were willing to carefully limit himself to these small portions, it still wouldn't be a good idea for him to "trade away" potatoes every day to make room for a sweet dessert. The dessert has no significant nutritional value, whereas potatoes have complex carbohydrate, potassium, and fiber. Still, it's reasonable to eat desserts occasionally, and having the freedom to have treats makes for a greater willingness to stick to a meal plan.

This trading one food for another may explain why your friend or family member with diabetes has claimed to be staying on their meal plan when you thought he or she was "cheating." The person may very well have been within the guidelines set by the dietitian or physician.

The Exchange List Doesn't Predict a Food's Effect on Blood Sugar Perfectly

The amount of carbohydrate in a food is not the only thing that influences blood sugar. We now know that some foods from different exchange lists that have different amounts of carbohydrate have a similar effect on blood sugar (such as carrots from the vegetable list and potatoes from the starch list).

The system of categorizing foods according to how quickly and how far they raise blood sugar is called the *Glycemic Index*. The Glycemic Index shows that white and wheat bread raises the blood sugar higher in three hours than does ice cream. And that regular potatoes raise it higher than sweet potatoes.

Most people with diabetes don't rely much on the glycemic index to pick isolated foods because they rarely eat a food by itself. For example, they don't usually eat bread alone—they eat it as part of a sandwich or with a meal. Also, an individual's reaction to a carbohydrate is just that—individual. So people with diabetes, by testing their blood after eating, can learn from experience what foods raise their blood sugars and avoid them or eat them in small amounts with other foods.

What Form a Food Is in, Matters

The greatest practical help of the research that resulted in the Glycemic Index is that we now know that the form the food is in makes a difference. It seems that the more pureed the food is, the quicker it is absorbed. Cooking also speeds up the transformation to sugar, as does eating a food on an empty stomach. In short, eating a raw chunk of food (like an apple) with a meal will raise blood sugar less than eating a cooked, pureed food (like applesauce) by itself.

Salt

Salt is not bad for everybody. Surprised to hear that? Most kidneys are very good at regulating the amount of salt and water that stays in our bodies.[6] Fortunately, about 70 percent of us have kidneys that do a good job. The other 30 percent of the population saves too much sodium. Since the body works best with a certain concentration of sodium, if there is too much, the kidneys try to dilute it by making less urine and retaining more water. More water in the blood vessels, means more pressure against

---

[6] Salt is part sodium and part chloride but the part of salt that is related to water retention is sodium.

the sides of those vessels, causing increasing blood pressure. Sometimes the body retains so much water that the ankles and even the whole body can swell. This swelling is called "edema." High blood pressure and edema cause the heart to work harder to push that volume of fluid around. Also, if you remember from Chapter 7 on complications, high blood pressure is bad for the kidneys and bad for the eyes.

But for most of us, if our kidneys take care of the sodium and water and we don't have a problem with edema, why do we have to limit the salt in our diets? We don't *have* to. On the other hand, we don't need all that salt, either. We'd get all we needed from healthy foods if we never picked up a salt shaker the rest of our lives. And we can't count on the kidneys to do a good job forever. As we age they lose more and more of their ability to regulate salt and fluid.

High blood pressure is almost always symptomless so you'd only find out that it was high after it was checked. Because high blood pressure is often associated with fluid retention, it might mean that your kidneys were not regulating salt well.

Cutting down on salt, then, is not required for most diabetics or for most nondiabetics. It is, though, for someone with high blood pressure, congestive heart failure, cirrhosis of the liver, kidney disease, and for people taking certain medications like steroids, for example.

The best advice is to cut down on salt. People who have given up salt on their doctors' orders usually say that in a week they find canned foods and other highly salty, processed food too salty for their newly-trained taste buds. They don't miss the salt at all.

It is such an easy vice to get rid of, please think about making this positive change for yourself and your loved ones, with or without diabetes.

Fiber

Fiber is a food ingredient that influences blood sugar--and a lot more. Its benefits include:
- increasing the effectiveness of insulin
- delaying and smoothing the adsorption of sugars from the digestive tract
- lowering cholesterol and trigliceride levels
- lowering blood presure
- promoting weight loss (by making you feel full longer after eating)
- helping prevent colon, breast, and ovarian cancers
- helping prevent constipation, diverticulosis and hemorrhoids

Fiber is available only from plant foods. There is no fiber in meat, for example, no matter how chewy it is.

There are two types of fiber, insoluble and soluble. Insoluble fiber is present in whole wheat products, wheat and corn bran, and many vegetables. It's called insoluble because it holds on to water but it doesn't dissolve in it. These qualities help it move foods through the digestive tract faster, reducing exposure of the intestines' walls to cancer-causing agents in food. It's ability to attract water into the digestive tract also softens the stools and helps prevent constipation.

Soluble fiber, the type found in dried beans and peas, oats, barley, and many fruits and vegetables (such as apples, oranges, and carrots) dissolves in water. It becomes like a gel and slows down the whole process of absorption through the wall of the intestine. Glucose, is also more slowly absorbed in the presence of soluble fiber so the usual rise of the blood glucose level, especially right after meals, is more gradual. Thus, soluble fiber can help keep blood sugar levels more stable. Soluble fiber also decreases blood cholesterol and other blood fats.

Most North Americans don't eat enough fiber. We generally average only about 11 grams of fiber a day instead of 25–35 grams many experts recommend. It's not hard to get enough fiber when we eat mostly vegetables, fruits, and foods made from whole grains (all rich in one or both types of fiber). But since we don't, the easiest way to get a lot of fiber is to start the day with a bowl of high fiber cereal. Not all cereals are good sources of fiber (check the number of fiber grams under Total Carbohydrate on the label). Cereals with double-digit amounts of fiber grams per serving are good sources--cereals with "high fiber" or "bran" in their names may not be. The following cereals are arranged in order from those most concentrated in fiber to those with very little.

Fiber in 100 calories of Breakfast Cereal

	grams of total fiber		grams of total fiber
All Bran Extra Fiber	28	Grape Nuts	3
Fiber One	22	Shredded Wheat	3
Oat Bran	6	35% Fruit Muesli	3
Fiberwise	5	Frosted Mini Wheats	3
Healthy Valley High Fiber O's	5	Oat Meal	3
Raisin Bran	5	Multi-grain Cheerios	2
Shredded Wheat 'N Bran	4	Corn Flakes	1
Fruit & Fiber	4	Special K	0.6
Total Wheat	4	Wheaties	0.5

Food That's Good for People with Diabetes Is Good for Everybody

There are more similarities than differences in what we should be eating and what someone with diabetes should be eating. Instead of setting diabetics apart as a deprived group that can't eat what we eat because they are sick, we should be looking at them as models of how *to eat so as not* to get sick.

What nutritionists recommend for:

People *with* diabetes	People *without* diabetes
Low fat, especially low saturated fat	Low fat, especially low saturated fat
High fiber	High fiber
Moderate protein	Moderate protein
High complex carbohydrates	High complex carbohydrates
Low concentrated sugar	Low concentrated sugar
Low salt (possibly)	Low salt (possibly)
Calories to maintain a sensible weight	Calories to maintain a sensible weight

There's no difference in these two lists because eating low fat, high fiber, moderate protein, high carbohydrate (but not the ones with low nutritional value like sugar), possibly low salt, and just enough calories to maintain a sensible weight, is the prescription for preventing numerous diseases. The number one cause of death in North America is still heart and cardiovascular disease. Nursing homes are full of people disabled by strokes. High cholesterol and high levels of fat in the blood, plus high blood pressure exacerbated by high salt diets are implicated in heart disease and strokes. Colon cancer is more prevalent in people who eat high fat, low fiber diets. But it doesn't have to happen, at least not at the relatively young ages that heart attacks and strokes and cancer are felling us.

The sensible diabetic and all health-conscious nondiabetics should be eating the same foods! So find a diabetic who is taking good care of himself and eat what he eats!

Chapter 11
Inviting Someone With Diabetes To Your Home For a Meal

Have you ever invited someone with diabetes to your home for a meal and then felt uncertainty and panic, wondering what to serve? My neighbor Beth came to me with that problem. Her brother was bringing his girlfriend, Patty, over for the Fourth of July family barbecue and Beth was panicky about what to serve.

Beth doesn't need to wriggle out of hosting the party, or prepare two menus, or buy everything in the dietetic section of her supermarket.

In this chapter we'll discuss what questions to ask your guest with diabetes before meal plans are finalized. There are samples of good and not-so-good menus, and examples of ways to reduce sugar and fat. Suggestions on where to find recipes and other specific helps round out this guide.

To get back to helping Beth, she will feel a lot more confident if she calls Patty to find out what Patty can eat and when she needs to eat. In fact, that's the first thing you should do if you want to avoid misunderstandings.

Ask If Timing is Important

The first question you should ask is, "Do you need to eat at a certain time?" Once you have agreed on a time for dinner, ask, "Is it important that we stay with that exact time or do you have some leeway?" Time is usually important for someone taking insulin once or twice a day and may also be for someone taking oral medication to lower blood sugar. Briefly this is because these medications are taken in advance with the expectation that food will be eaten to coincide with their peak action times. Without food, blood sugar can get too low.

People who control their diabetes solely by diet and exercise have fewer constraints placed on their eating schedule. At the other end of the treatment spectrum are those who inject insulin with every meal and those who wear an insulin pump that gives insulin whenever it's needed. They don't have to match their food to their insulin schedule because they're matching their insulin to their food schedule. They take insulin twenty to thirty minutes before the food will be served, so a delay they know about in time to hold off on their insulin is not any more of an issue to them than your stomach growling is to you.

Patty's answer to Beth about this question was that it would be easiest for her to eat between 5:00 and 6:00 since this was her usual evening meal hour. She added that she could make some adjustments if that wasn't convenient.

Beth was glad she'd asked since it was no problem to schedule the dinner for around 5:30. She was especially glad because Patty sounded very pleasantly surprised that Beth had bothered, and Patty's "thank you" was nice to hear.

Ask About Food Restrictions

In this day of allergies and diets for all kinds of medical conditions, from asthma to ulcers, it is a kindness to ask any guest if they have any special food needs you should consider in planning the meal.

If you asked a hundred people with diabetes what they could and couldn't eat, you would likely get fifty different answers. You could hear anything from, "Don't fuss, I can eat the same food you can," to "I can eat anything low-fat that doesn't have sugar in it."

A person with diabetes *may not* be able to eat:
> Desserts made with sugar
> Foods made with honey, corn syrup, or barbecue sauce
> Regular maple syrup, jams, and jellies
> Foods high in protein (meat, fish, and dairy products)
> Foods high in fat (butter, margarine, fatty meats,
> mayonnaise, cheese, cream, salad dressing, etc.)

A person with diabetes *may* be able to eat:
> Desserts made with artificial sweeteners (Equal, Sunette,
> Sweet 1, SugarTwin, and saccharine)
> Desserts made with sugar (in small quantities)
> Vegetables cooked with little or no sugar or fat
> Salads with low-fat dressing
> Syrups and jams made with artificial sweeteners (just because it
> says "Lite" or "no added sugar" is not automatically OK—
> ask or read the label carefully)
> Bread
> Foods that are broiled, steamed or baked without added fat
> Pasta, rice, and potatoes without fatty sauces and toppings
> Lean meats, poultry, and fish

Again, the variety of responses you may get are a result of different treatment plans and different goals. Treatment can change over time, too, so you'll want to get current information. For example, the relative you invite today may need to be very rigid about food choices because of the need to maintain a certain blood sugar or protect his kidneys or keep blood pressure down. A few months ago, though, he may not have had the same motivation or the same medical necessity.

Imagine, though, your friend or relative with diabetes at a get-together where the only thing served that he or she can eat is tossed salad or veggies with no dressing, and the only thing to drink without sugar or alcohol is water.

This could happen if the menu was one of these:

Menu #1: A Barbecue
Chips and onion dip
Barbecued ribs
Potato salad
Coleslaw
Macaroni salad
Corn bread
Tossed salad
Ice cream sundaes
Regular soda
Wine and beer

Menu #2: Dinner for Company
Cream of mushroom soup
Prime rib roast
Creamed onions
Twice-baked potatoes
Buttered broccoli
Raw vegetable plate
Hot rolls
Apple pie
Wine
Coffee[1]

In Menu #1, the person who is watching fat and cholesterol intake is left with the tossed salad, and that may have to be with little or no dressing unless the host provides a low-fat salad dressing. All the other salads are high in fat from mayonnaise, and the corn bread contains con-

---

[1] Plain coffee and tea do not have calories or raise blood sugar. However, coffee creamers are high in sugar and fat and flavored gourmet coffee blends may be also.

siderable fat and sugar. The chips, dip, and ribs are all fatty so they're not a good idea (except for tiny tastes). There's no sugar-free soda, so the only safe beverages are one glass of wine or beer (if the calories in the wine or beer are not a problem) and water.

Menu #2 contains lots of fat and a dessert high in both fat and sugar. For careful people, only the raw vegetables and a hot roll or two plus coffee can be eaten in normal quantities without guilt or problems. Everything else has to be taken in very small portions or skipped.

Here are some of the comments I hear from people with diabetes about choices when eating with friends and family:

"It would be thoughtful if they'd have things I can have as well, such as diet soda."

"Tell me if it's made with sugar or other sweeteners and, if so, how much. I don't like surprises."

"I wish people knew how much I appreciated them offering alternative desserts."

What Should You Serve?

What's the answer? I recommended to my neighbor Beth that she start with a heart-healthy menu that would be good for everyone, including herself. (Alternatively, she could keep the fatty foods and add a couple of extra items to the menu that are low in fat and sugar).

For example, at the barbecue where Menu #1 is to be served, Beth could have skinless chicken breast or some of the new low-fat hot dogs like Hormel's (97 percent fat-free) Light and Lean Franks. She could have plain bread or rolls (most have little or no fat). For dessert she could serve a fruit salad with whipped topping or ice cream on the side. Offering a selection of salad dressings, including a low-fat or nonfat variety, is a considerate touch. At my urging, Beth also decided to have sugar-free soda, including one with no caffeine, since this is also an ingredient many people try to avoid, for reasons unrelated to diabetes.

Although Patty would have enough choices with the preceding changes, I proposed that Beth try to serve a meal that would be healthier for everyone—for Patty, for Beth's sixtyish parents and in-laws, for Beth and her sister and brother who have been battling their weight for years, for her husband with the borderline high cholesterol, and for her kids.

This is the menu that Beth created and which I heartily approved:

A Better Barbecue Menu

Raw vegetable platter with low-fat dip
Marinated chicken breast kabobs
Foil-grilled Idaho or sweet potatoes
Sliced tomatoes and cucumbers
Fresh fruit salad (unsweetened)
Whipped topping (on the side)
Sugar-free lemonade or diet soda
Regular soda
Wine and beer

Alternatives to Menu #2 include roast turkey or baked or broiled fish instead of the prime rib, baked potatoes with sour cream and butter on the side, unbuttered vegetables, and a low-fat, low-sugar dessert such as a chiffon pie made with artificial sweetener (the *very* careful can eat only the filling and leave the crust) or a commercial sugar-free dessert like Dreyer's Sugar Free Frozen Dietary Dairy Dessert.

A Better Dinner for Company Menu

Minestrone soup
Broiled salmon with lemon slices
Hungarian green beans (recipe in Appendix)
Baked potatoes with toppings on the side
Mixed green salad with low-fat dressing
Dinner roll
Mixed berry cup with sugar-free vanilla
    frozen dairy dessert
Sugar-free soda or mineral water with
    lemon slice
Wine
Coffee and tea

Beverages

Sugar-free sodas are very popular and will be welcome to most diabetics. Beware when shopping, however. There are some flavored sparkling waters and clear sodas that look as though they're sugar-free but aren't. They are sweetened with high-fructose corn syrup. Many have as almost as much sugar and calories as regular soda pop. *Check the label carefully* for ingredients and look for a drink that is *artificially* sweetened.

Alcohol is another tricky beverage. It can lead to severely low blood sugars if drunk without a meal or if drunk to excess even with food. (For more about the low blood sugar dangers of alcohol see Chapter 12 on dining out).

In addition to the safety issue, alcohol has a surprisingly high number of calories, almost as many as fat. One and a half ounces of hard liquor, 4 ounces of wine, or 12 ounces of beer each have the equivalent of two fat exchanges or 90 calories from the alcohol portion alone. Wine and beer have still more calories from the carbohydrate they also contain.

Yet another disadvantage of alcohol is that it can help people forget their diets and pile on the wrong foods.

Except for preventing someone from drinking to excess, which is truly dangerous, a considerate host or hostess may offer, but should never push, alcohol.

Dessert

Don't automatically include a recipe or a commercial product because of broad terms like "diabetic dessert."[2] Many recipes and diabetic foods are geared toward the younger, insulin-dependent diabetic who may not have a weight problem and who may only be concerned about limiting sugars and other carbohydrates.

Most diabetic desserts have almost as many calories as ordinary sweets. All the fat has been left in the candies, cookies, and cake mixes, and it's the fat that primarily raises the calorie count.

Since three-quarters of the people with diabetes need to watch their calorie and fat intake as much as their sugar, high-fat commercial foods and recipes that call for a 1/2 cup or more of butter or cream cheese are not acceptable even if they are artificially sweetened.

This again emphasizes the importance of asking what your guest's restrictions are and not making assumptions.

---

[2] See Chapter 10 for more about diabetic products in the supermarket.

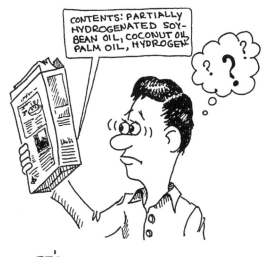

IT'S IMPORTANT TO READ LABELS
TO KNOW WHAT YOU'RE SERVING.

How to Reduce Sugar in Foods

Chances are good, though, that you'll be asked to use little or no sugar at least in part of the menu. That's trickier than you might imagine, since lots of substances are chemically sugars but are not known by that name.

Any sweetener that has calories can raise blood sugar. These caloric sweeteners have 4 calories a gram. That doesn't sound like much, but for ordinary granulated sugar, that translates into 770 calories per cup.

Here are some other names for sugar:

Molasses	Raw sugar	Treacle	Turbinado
Brown sugar	Honey	Refiners' syrup	

Some people claim that because these sugars are not refined, they provide valuable nutrients. The amount of any nutrients, however, is so small that calories from any of these sweeteners should be considered empty calories.

Another group of sweeteners that have calories includes sorbitol, mannitol, dulcitol, and xylitol. These artificial sweeteners are absorbed more slowly into the blood than sugar and therefore may cause a less dramatic blood sugar rise, especially in someone who is not completely dependent on injections for insulin. However, they tend to cause bloating and diarrhea when eaten in large quantities. (The amount in a package of Tic Tacs or two sugar-free hard candies can cause discomfort).

Lactose is a sugar put in milk by the cow. It is a natural and caloric sweetener. This milk sugar is why sugar is listed in the "Nutrition Facts" label on every dairy product in the section titled, "Total Carbohydrate."

Fructose is a natural sugar commonly found in fruits. It doesn't raise the blood sugar rapidly in well-controlled diabetes, but it has calories and must be counted as a carbohydrate. Note that while it doesn't raise blood sugar as rapidly, it does raise it, especially in people whose blood sugar is generally too high. Fructose is found in many dietetic products and commercial baked goods. There is no significant advantage to using fructose or the fruit juices commonly called for in older diabetic cookbooks. Your body can't really tell the difference between the sugar from an apple (or other fruit) and the sugar from a beet or cane.

Fructose has another problem. Studies have shown that fructose, along with table sugar, can contribute to higher LDL cholesterol (the bad kind) and triglyceride levels.[3] Since people with diabetes are already more prone to high cholesterol and triglycerides and because the higher these blood fats are, the greater their risk of having a heart attack or stroke, anything that contributes to raising these must be used in moderation.

Syrups and other forms of glucose are common sweeteners in baked goods and commercial products. The syrup you've probably heard of most, is corn syrup. Here's a list of the more common varieties of glucose you may see in the ingredients list of a product:

Glucose	Corn syrup	Rice syrup
Maltose	Potato syrup	Barley syrup
Carob powder	Tapioca syrup	Dextrin
Dextrose	Sorghum syrup	Starch syrup

Food labels list ingredients in decreasing order of their quantity in the product. Try to steer clear of foods that have one of the above sugars or syrups as the first ingredient. Also avoid those that list several caloric sweeteners, no matter where they are on the list of ingredients. Even small amounts add up—some manufacturers use several different sweeteners to make it seem as though the total amount of sweeteners is less than it really is. They do this by using small enough quantities of each so that they appear lower in the list of ingredients.

---

[3] Fructose can be used in small quantities but not as a substitute for granulated sugar in recipes calling for generous amounts of sugar.

Some sweeteners that have no calories and that do not raise blood sugar are:

> Equal (aspartame or NutraSweet)
> Sweet One (acesulfame potassium or acesulfame-K)
> Saccharin (SugarTwin, Sweet'N Low, etc.)
> Cyclamates (not available in the U.S.)

Artificial Sweetners Have Limitations

You can substitute noncaloric or artificial sweeteners for sugar, honey, and syrups in some recipes. Equal, however, does not withstand prolonged heating, so it cannot be used as a cake, pie, or baked bean ingredient. It is able to withstand the heat of boiling water added to gelatin, though, or it can be added after a dish is cooked. It does not add the texture that is needed in some baked goods, which sugar provides in addition to sweetness.

For baking you can try SugarTwin, which has a bulking agent added for texture and saccharin for sweetness. The good news is that saccharin can be used in baking. The bad news with SugarTwin and other saccharine products is that the saccharin in them can leave a bitter aftertaste.

Sweet One can be used in baking. It does not have a bulking agent like SugarTwin, so the manufacturers recommend replacing only part of the sugar with Sweet One to preserve the texture.

All of the sweeteners require smaller amounts if two or more are combined. That means you could use SugarTwin and Sweet One, instead of sugar, and reduce the total amount that the products' sugar equivalent charts call for. If you're creative, try this mixing to get the best qualities of each sweetener. Artificial sweetners substituted for sugar can enable a beverage or gelatin dessert to be carbohydrate and calorie free. Baked goods are not so "fortunate." For example, a typical blueberry muffin has four sources of carbohydrate: flour, sugar, blueberries, and milk.

As you can see, even if you substituted all the sugar with an artificial sweetener, and didn't mind that the muffin would be dry and gummy, you'd only reduce the carbohydrate by 25%. The flour is a much more significant source of blood-sugar-raising carbohydrate, but until someone invents artificial flour, baked goods will continue to be large sources of carbohydrate even when made with artificial sweetener.

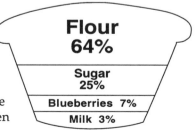

Sugar in Moderation

Sugar does not have to be completely avoided. For many years, it was believed that simple sugar, like honey or table sugar, is responsible for quicker and higher rises in blood sugar than complex carbohydrates (starches) such as rice and potatoes. Recent research, however, suggests that the difference is not very significant.

So it is the total amount of carbohydrate (all the sugars and all the starches) that should be considered **in a meal**. Whether the diabetic gets the carbohydrate from bread, beans, or maple syrup will not significantly change the high point of his or her blood sugar after the meal.

In theory this means that a diabetic could eat a few spoonfuls of granulated sugar instead of some or all of the bread, potatoes, pasta, milk, fruit, or any other food that contains carbohydrate. Notice the word "instead." No one can eat the usual amount of carbohydrate at mealtime **and** add sugar. The result would be high blood sugar. Plus, the more nutritious bread, milk, etc. would have to be sacrificed to leave a carbohydrate "ration" for the sugar.

This fairly new idea is being greeted with mixed feelings. Some diabetics say they are quite sensitive to simple sugar and feel that they are better off without it.

Others welcome the greater freedom that "trading" can mean to them. It means they can eat a slice of birthday cake or a candy bar if they omit an equivalent amount of some other carbohydrate (and maybe fat too).

The disadvantage of eating a candy bar or cake instead of a more nutritious food is that they would be trading empty sugar calories (and probably lots of fat) for a serving of fiber, vitamins, minerals, and other nutrients.

Another problem is that sugar is not called a concentrated sweet for nothing. That means that it doesn't take much sugar to add up to a lot of a less concentrated carbohydrate.

For example, here's what a diabetic would have to trade away to eat just one tablespoon of sugar:

1 dinner roll (or)
1 slice bread (or)
1 glass milk (or)
3 cups popcorn

Each of these foods is a lot of nutritious food to give up for a food with one tablespoon of sugar. And if you consider that a single slice of chocolate cake with chocolate frosting has about 3 3/4 tablespoons of sugar, that's equal to 11 1/4 cups of popcorn or, more realistically, 3 cups of popcorn, 1 slice bread, 1 glass of milk, and a dinner roll!

Knowing the amount of sugar per serving would be a help to your guest in deciding what and how much to choose from several carbohydrates to equal his or her total carbohydrate ration. You can help your guest with diabetes keep a normal blood sugar and still enjoy the food you serve.

The easiest way to know the amount of carbohydrate in a dish is to use recipes that include this information. See Resources for some good cookbooks.

How to Reduce Fat in Foods

The most common sources of fat in food are dairy products, meats, and oils used in frying and dressings.

Milk and milk products can be a high or low in fat. Here are some dairy products that have little or no fat:

Nonfat (skim) milk	Fat-free buttermilk	Evaporated skim milk
Nonfat dry milk	Plain, nonfat yogurt	1% lowfat milk
Nonfat sour cream	Nonfat or lowfat cottage cheese	

You may have wondered why cheese is not on the list. That's because non-diet cheese is so high in fat that it is considered more like meat. In diabetes nutrition guides meats and cheeses are divided into high-fat, medium-fat, and lean meat groups depending on their fat content.

Most meats fall into the medium-fat category. Prime cuts of beef and almost all cheeses, such as American, Blue, Cheddar, Monterey, and Swiss are in the high-fat group.

Your best choices will come from the very lean or lean meat and very lean or lean meat substitutes listed here:

Canadian bacon	Ham (fresh or boiled)	
Chicken	Lunch meat (97% fat-free)	Tenderloin
Chipped beef	Oysters	Tuna (fresh or
Cornish hen	Parmesan cheese	canned in
Diet cheese	Rabbit	water)
Fish	Shellfish	Turkey
Flank steak	Sirloin (lean)	Venison

Egg yolks have enough fat in them to put whole eggs into the medium-fat meat group. Yolks are also high in cholesterol, so they should only be eaten, at most, three times a week. There are some healthy ways to use egg whites, however. Here are some low-fat options:

Egg whites
Egg substitutes with less than 55 calories per 1/4 cup
> (Some egg substitutes are made of only egg whites and coloring, whereas others have added vegetable oil. You'll need to read the label on the carton for the fat and calorie content)

The occasional whole egg should be poached, boiled or "fried" in a non-stick pan with Pam or other cooking spray.

Meat Portions
In addition to choosing a lean meat or lean meat substitute, you need to know how much is an allowable portion for a diabetic. You'll probably consider diabetic portions very small compared to what you're used to. Again, the usual diabetic meat portion is 3 ounces, which is about the size of a pack of playing cards. Some examples of 3-ounce meat portions are:

> 1/2 chicken breast
> 1 unbreaded fish fillet
> 3/4 cup canned tuna in water
> 5 medium canned sardines
> 1 small hamburger patty

Meat Preparation Suggestions

1. To cook meat, don't fry, instead bake, broil, boil, roast, or grill.
2. Trim off visible fat before and after cooking.
3. Do not add flour, bread crumbs, or coating mixes (they absorb fat).
4. Use a nonstick pan and nonstick spray to brown or "fry."
5. Cook meat or poultry on a rack so the fat will drain off.
6. Do not serve with gravy or sauce.

Miscellaneous Sources of Fat

Other sources of fat besides meat, eggs, cheese, and milk products are foods rich in vegetable fats. These include:

Avocado	Nondairy coffee creamer	Olives
Coconut	Peanut butter	Seeds (sunflower,
Margarine	Vegetable shortening	pumpkin and,
Nuts	Vegetable oil	pine nuts)

None of the above foods has cholesterol because all of them are plant products and cholesterol comes only from animals. But they are all high-fat and some are 100 percent fat, so they are easily transformed into excess body fat. By limiting them as much as possible in the food you serve — you will be kind to yourself as well.

In addition to trying low-fat cooking techniques and new recipes, be on the lookout for new products in your market. The food industry regularly launches new fat-free and low-fat foods that make healthy eating increasingly sacrifice-free.

Consider Serving-Size

What is healthy and what is not, is not only determined by the ingredient list. When you shop look at the number of servings and the size of servings the product has. If you just look at the number of calories per serving, you could be fooled. Even potato chips don't seem bad at 145 calories per ounce. Most of us can afford a 145-calorie splurge a day. But if you notice that the bag contains 12 ounces and the manufacturer says a serving is 1 ounce, you know that 145 calories is 1/12th the package! I don't know about you, but for *me* a normal serving size of potato chips would be 1/2 bag or 6 servings. Multiplying 145 by 6 equals 870 calories! So I don't buy or serve potato chips. Serving sizes printed on packages are notoriously skimpy. You need to estimate what *you* consider a realistic serving and calculate whether or not it is still a fat/calorie/sugar bargain.

What Should You Say
If the Person With Diabetes Takes a "Bad" Food?

One of the most common complaints I hear from people with diabetes is that nonmedical people without diabetes try to point out what they shouldn't be eating. Often the advice givers are wrong, especially if they are operating from the mistaken idea that no one with diabetes should ever eat sugar.

As has been mentioned, *small to moderate amounts* of sugar or honey or other blood sugar raising sweeteners actually may not be bad, provided they are eaten with a balanced meal and are calculated within the allowances for carbohydrate, protein, and fat for that meal.

So, raised eyebrows, shocked looks, shaking heads, and even a whispered, "Should you be eating that?" are generally infuriating to people with diabetes. When I asked what they do when someone tells them what to eat, they said:

> "It depends who is telling me. If it is family, I feel it is a direct challenge to me, so I many times want to do the opposite." (Laura, 43)

"I do the opposite. I don't like others (parents, friends, etc.) controlling my diabetes. I have to live with it, they don't. They don't know what a diabetic goes through." (Samantha, 14)

"It depends on who is talking. If it's my doctor, she knows what she is talking about. If it's a friend or someone else's parent, I ignore them." (Megan, 13)

"Usually those who comment know very little about the disease and usually are overweight and should be on a diet and watch what they eat themselves!" (anonymous)

"I don't want reminders." (Joan, 29)

"When my husband criticizes a poor eating choice (nuts or cream, for instance), I bristle, but I know his criticism is warranted so the immediate effect is resentment, but the delayed effect is that it reinforces my resolve to avoid such foods as regular parts of my diet." (Elsa, 56)

Maybe your observation will have the long-term, positive effect that Elsa's husband's criticism has with her. But, judging from the responses I've gotten, it's more likely that you will irritate someone into doing just the opposite of what you're advising.

In short, what people with diabetes have asked me to tell you is that they will take care of it themselves. They will fill their plates or not, they will eat everything they've taken, or not, and they will eat cake or not. Until you have their level of knowledge about diabetes in general and their own diabetes in particular, you should not be making any but the most diplomatic suggestions and maybe not even those.

You want to help, though, so if you can't say things like, "Should you be eating that?" what can you do that they won't take wrong? Read on.

How to Help

In the area of food, the biggest help you can be to someone who has diabetes is to not sabotage their meal plan. I'm sure that would not be your intent, but it happens.

Mrs. Clark was an elderly widow from the South. She belonged to a church my diabetic friend Bob joined. Mrs. Clark loved to bake but she didn't get a chance to do it much after her husband died. He used to praise her pecan pies to the skies and she missed that so she baked for every church event she could. She would hover over her pies and urge people to eat, and then urge them to eat some more. Of course they complimented her on her pecan pie (deservedly), while she beamed.

It wasn't enough to get ten or fifteen people to eat her pies, though. She wanted my friend Bob to "eat up" too. When he tried refusing, she looked sad. He tried taking only a taste, but when he wouldn't eat a whole piece, she thought he didn't like her pie and was crushed. It didn't make any difference when he said he had diabetes. Her rejoinder was, "Oh, but it's only this once." Since Bob knew that a 430-calorie piece of pecan pie with 24 grams of fat and 52 grams of carbohydrate (which is more than he usually gets in his whole lunch!) was going to send his blood sugar soaring, he stood firm.

Because he didn't do the easy thing and eat the pie to please Mrs. Clark, he was able to be tolerant of her efforts. But consider what his opinion of her, and himself as well, would have been if he had eaten the slice of pecan pie and found his blood sugar double or triple normal when he checked it later.

Bob is likely to meet Mrs. Clark or someone like her again. One tack he, and you, can take is to find something else to praise in people whose need for others to appreciate their cooking is at odds with the diabetic's food needs. Your voice, added to his, can make a difference to people like Mrs. Clark. I wouldn't give up trying to educate her a little about diabetes, either—she might decide to try her hand at low-fat, sugar-free desserts as a new challenge.

Instead of risking being a Mrs. Clark by having only pie or some other unhealthy old standby at your dinner, how about having fresh fruit available or a low-fat, artificially sweetened dessert that your family member or friend can have without guilt and without blood sugar elevations?

To find recipes for healthy dishes look in Recipes at the back of this book. Also try your library or bookstore for recently published cookbooks, the newer the better. Books written in the last ten years will give calorie and other nutritional information *plus* use available ingredients, including some new and improved products. Or ask your diabetic friends if they have a favorite dish they have been yearning for. You won't go wrong with *their* recipe.

When you serve your special recipe, though, don't make an issue of the fact that you went out of your way to produce this healthy dessert especially for your diabetic cousin Joan. First, you won't be alerting people that it's good for them, which might make them expect it to taste bad. But more importantly, Joan won't be embarrassed by having her

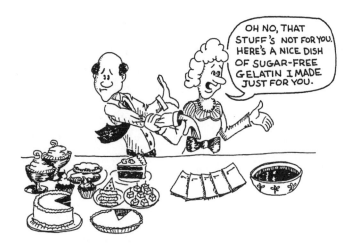

different needs advertised. You and Joan need be the only ones who know what a saint you are. Being singled out for special attention (and notoriety) is not welcomed. One of my friends was mortified at a dinner party to have the hostess bring her her very own plate of food especially prepared according to a diabetes cookbook. Imagine the work that that involved! Sadly, it was not appreciated. Lisa would have preferred to have had what everybody else had. If something was not on her meal plan, she could have had a tiny taste and left the rest.

If I seem to be contradicting myself, let me clarify what people with diabetes want. Either make everything low-fat, low-sugar, and so forth, or be ready to point out what the ingredients are *to everyone in ringing tones, or* to the person with diabetes in a discrete way.

At my last buffet dinner party, I had little notes stuck to foods that said things like "fat-free bean dip" and "sugar-free" by the whipped topping and the pumpkin pie. It did the job but didn't look very elegant. A guest who is famous for her entertaining skills suggested that I put place cards in decorative holders and use them instead to identify the ingredients.

I know from experience that serving healthier foods can be more work. It is more time-consuming to choose, wash, cut up, and display a tray of veggies than to dump out a bag of chips and open a container of fatty sour cream dip. Anyone can take the easy way that is bad for people. After all, many of us have a file box full of recipes that are made with ingredients we shouldn't be using. You can be different and be asked for your recipes. Compiling a file of healthy food that tastes good is the challenge of today's cook.

Chapter 12
Dining Out With Someone With Diabetes

John, who has insulin-dependent diabetes, told me about getting an invitation to go out after work. Since he was new in the office, he was pleased to be included in the group. But their plans caused him some concern. This is how the conversation went:

SUSAN: John, a bunch of us from accounting and personnel are planning to go out to dinner after work. Would you like to join us?

JOHN: I sure would, what time will we eat and where?

SUSAN: Oh, we always go to the Big Drinks Lounge for two-dollar drinks at happy hour. We decide later where and when to eat dinner—that is, if we don't feel full after pretzels and peanuts. If we go to a restaurant afterwards, it's usually to Gus's Grease Garden or the Stupendous Steak.

Why is John concerned about these plans? What's wrong with cocktails before dinner, a to-be-decided-later dinner time, and the restaurant choices? In this chapter we'll also discuss why even a little alcohol without a meal can be dangerous for someone with diabetes, how easy it is to confuse a low blood sugar with overindulgence in alcohol, and why mealtimes need to be on schedule. You'll learn the right questions to ask a diabetic and how to help others who don't have diabetes understand why keeping to a timetable for meals is not just a whim. By supporting the person with diabetes you'll lessen the likelihood that he or she will fail to ask the server about ingredients and cooking methods and keep mum about an unhealthy restaurant choice. For example, he might be tempted to jettison his meal plan to "be one of the gang." Choosing the right restaurant and making the right menu selections can help the person with diabetes stay on a healthy diet.

As we discussed in Chapter 10, what a diabetic eats is an important part of his or her treatment plan. In general, eating healthily means reducing fat, calories, sodium, and sugar, and increasing vegetables, grains, and fresh fruits.

You Too Can Eat Wisely

I do hope that you too, are making some of these healthier choices for yourself, at least when you are with this special person. Even if you don't have an immediate medical reason to restrict your fat or salt or sugar, doing so will benefit you in the long run. You will be setting a good example, will make your friend or family member with diabetes feel less different, and you'll save them from casting yearning looks at what is on your plate and feeling deprived.

A bonus for you is that you, too, will eat healthier food that looks and tastes good.

Alcohol and Diabetes

You might spare John some discomfort if you can help avoid the happy hour scene. The free hors d'oeuvres are almost invariably not healthy and the drinks are not a good idea for John either.

When a person with diabetes drinks alcohol his or her blood sugar can become too low, with serious consequences.

Low blood sugar is not only uncomfortable, it can cause falls and auto accidents, even without alcohol. Just as critical, however, is the potential for mistaking the symptoms of low blood sugar for being "under the influence." Symptoms of low blood sugar include poor coordination and slurred speech. Add another symptom, confusion, and you have someone who looks and acts like they're drunk. When any of us drink alcohol, our liver concentrates on processing the alcohol and stops providing us with the between-meal sugar that helps keep blood from getting too low.

If someone with diabetes is just left to "sleep it off," and nobody thinks to give juice or food, the consequences could be drastic. The insulin keeps working, there's no food intake, and without the liver's help to release emergency sugar because of the alcohol, the "sleep" could become permanent.

It is possible for a diabetic to drink a glass of wine with dinner because the food will keep the blood sugar from getting too low, so the reserve supply in the liver will not be needed. One or, at most, two drinks can be safely consumed—but only with a meal.

Even if the diabetic eats while he or she is drinking, there is a limit to how long the food will maintain the blood sugar level when more than one or two drinks are consumed. What happens when the food stops working, but the liver is still "off duty," working on the alcohol? What if the result is a very low blood sugar at 3 a.m. with no one around to observe it and do what's necessary?[1]

There is no safe way for a person with diabetes to drink a lot. Moderation is essential, and for someone with diabetes, moderation means one or two drinks.

---

[1] See Chapter 8 for more about low blood sugar symptoms and treatment.

A final point about alcoholic drinks is to remember that they're fattening—almost as fattening as pats of butter. Most people with Type II diabetes are trying to lose weight, and the addition of drinks to a meal means excess calories. Hopefully, the person trying to lose weight will choose a diet soda or water instead of wine, beer, or whiskey. Twisting the person's arm to join you in an alcoholic beverage is another push towards loss of control.

Scheduling A Time

The same concern with mealtime that's important when you invite someone to your home to eat, is important when dining out. Again, ask the person with diabetes, "Once we agree on a time for dinner, is it important that we stay with that time?"[2]

Scheduling includes knowing if the restaurant you're considering is still in business, checking the hours it's open, making reservations, if appropriate, and knowing the traffic will let you get there within an hour of the diabetic's expected dinnertime.

If your car breaks down or there's an extreme road condition that gets you stuck in traffic, John will manage with the snacks he usually carries, or he'll tell you if you need to get him some soda or food. My point is that everyone will be happier if the *preventable* inconveniences are eliminated.

Choosing The Restaurant

Dining out means no one in the party has to do the cooking but *it doesn't relieve the planner from considering the kind of restaurant.* Any restaurant will have healthy and unhealthy menu choices. But certain types of restaurants will have more options for a health-conscious person with or without diabetes.

Chinese

Although Chinese restaurants have some less healthy items, such as fried egg rolls, fried wontons, butterfly shrimp, and sweet and sour pork, most dishes use the stir-fry method with little or no sugar and very little oil. You can even request that the "dry wok" cooking method be used. Numerous entrees are mainly vegetables, with only a little meat added for

---

[2] See Chapter 11 "Inviting Someone With Diabetes to Your Home for A Meal," for the reasons why this may be important.

flavor. Chinese restaurants have many healthy options, but you or some-one with diabetes still must ask what is deep-fried and what has sugar, at least until you have settled on some safe favorite dishes.

Thai, Vietnamese, Indian, and Japanese

Some good Asian cuisines, in addition to Chinese, are Indian, Thai, Viet-namese, and Japanese (skip the deep-fried tempura and opt for the sukiyaki, sushi, and vegetables). Most Thai dishes are stir-fried, steamed, boiled, or barbecued, but try to avoid duck, cashews, peanut sauce, co-conut milk—all extremely fatty—and the highly sugared iced tea.

Mexican

Although Mexican restaurants start out with some healthy ingredients like beans and salsa, they are famous for their deep-fried foods, cheese toppings, sour cream, avocado, and lard-laden tortillas. It's tough to eat healthily at a Mexican restaurant. It *can* be done by being very picky and creative, for example, by ordering a taco salad with no meat or avocado but lots of salsa. Have the cheese and sour cream served on the side, and leave them, along with the fried shell on the plate. And skip the nacho chips! See what I mean about being picky? Mexican restaurants make ordering significantly more difficult.

Fast Food

It used to be that fast-food restaurants had nothing for people who were trying to eat healthily. McDonald's now has the McLean Deluxe (skip the cheese) and salads, while almost every other fast food restaurant has some kind of *grilled (ask to be sure it's not fried)* chicken sandwich. To be really on track, you still have to scrape off some of the mayo and beware of fried anything. One of the best additions to their menus is the salad with low-fat dressing.

Ordering, for anyone concerned about fat, calories, sodium, or carbo-hydrates, has been made easier by the printed ingredient summaries many fast-food places now offer. You may have to ask for a copy, though, because they are not always displayed.

Coffee Shop Breakfast

Almost no combination or special on a breakfast menu is low in fat. Even if bacon, fried eggs, omelets, sausage, waffles, and French toast are skipped, it's hard to order healthily. Croissants have a buttery dough, muffins have lots of oil, and hash browns are just another name for fried potatoes.

Breakfast is best ordered from the side order section. There you and your friend can get oatmeal or cold cereal with nonfat milk, a fruit cup, and toast (butter on the side).

Alternatively, pancakes ordered without butter are relatively low in fat and most restaurants have sugar-free maple syrup for your friend with diabetes. There's nothing that says you can't have *your* pancakes with it too. You probably will not like it as well, but your willingness to try it and your ease at letting the waitress think *you're* different are good demonstrations of the fact that you two are a team. It also shows your friend or family member with diabetes what is available and how to get it if he or she doesn't already know.

Beware of healthy-sounding foods like yogurt, which in restaurants, is usually neither low-fat nor sugar-free, and granola, which is the fattiest cereal under the rising morning sun.

Sandwiches

Sandwiches can be lean or mean. At home, most of us make a sandwich with a teaspoon of mayonnaise per slice of bread, but restaurants often slather 1 to 1 1/2 *tablespoons* of mayo on their sandwiches. (One tablespoon of mayonnaise contains 100 calories and 11 grams of fat).

What goes between the bread makes a big difference, too. Here are some good and bad choices:

Low-Fat Sandwich Fillings	**High-Fat Sandwich Fillings**
Beef brisket	Cheese
Extra lean corned beef	Chicken salad with mayo
Extra lean pastrami	Cold cuts
Lean ham	Egg salad with mayo
Lean roast beef	Fried chicken patties
Roasted chicken breast	Fried fish
Roasted turkey breast	Hamburgers
Skinless grilled chicken	Salami
breast	Tuna salad with mayo

Last, but not least, portion size is important. Even if your diabetic friend orders a sandwich with turkey breast and lean roast beef, if it's a submarine sandwich it's probably large enough to feed two people. Perhaps you could agree to share.

Salads and Salad Bars

Salads can be a low-fat meal or side dish that supplies a large portion of vitamins and fiber-rich foods, or they can be loaded with fat. Worse, many times people who eat a salad for lunch feel so virtuous that they go overboard at dinner, sure that they have some calories in their "bank."

Here are just two examples of salads that are *not* low-fat:

Chef's salad (2 cups)   800 calories/65 grams fat
with cheese, boiled eggs,
roast beef, ham, and
turkey roll with a
creamy dressing)

Tossed salad (2 cups)   900 calories/70 grams fat
with bacon bits, cold
cuts, egg yolks, olives,
creamy pasta, potato
salad, and bleu cheese
dressing

Either one of these salads has more calories than a double bacon cheese-burger with a regular order of fries! Salad dressing alone can make a salad a high-fat food. The amount of dressing in a ladle at a normal salad bar holds 6 tablespoons, which alone can equal the fat and calories of a Big Mac. The salads above were calculated to have 4 tablespoons of dressing, or 300 calories' worth. That's still a lot of fat for something as "unspecial" as salad dressing.

Here's what to *skip* to keep a salad healthy:

Bacon bits	Macaroni salad
Cheese	Olives
Cold cuts	Potato salad
Croutons	Regular salad dressing
Egg yolks	Seeds
Fruit and Jello in	
whipped cream	

Since you are probably not holding the hand that holds the spoon, what can you do if your friend or relative with diabetes shovels on the grated cheddar and bacon bits? You can omit these from *your* salad and serve as a good role model. If you're lucky, you may find an opening to mention that you read that one scoop of potato salad made with mayonnaise has as many calories as one scoop of Breyer's regular chocolate ice cream. Maybe you will get a discussion going about hidden fat in foods and can plant some good ideas.

Buffets

Salad bars and smorgasbords have inspired a type of restaurant that can be good or bad: the buffet. It's theoretically possible to choose a wonderful variety of only healthy foods at a buffet. The problem is, can you and your friend or family member with diabetes resist the cinnamon rolls, corn bread, potatoes au gratin, pasta with cream sauce, carved roast beef, and the dessert table? Also, there's always the danger of overeating just to be sure you're getting your money's worth.

Generally, I recommend skipping the buffet restaurant because of its many temptations and because of the handicap its self-service places on communication. If you like the people you're with and you want to have a conversation, a buffet restaurant has serious drawbacks. At the start of dinner, no one is together because everyone is choosing their first plate of food. Later, someone will get up for more, taste it, and pronounce it good, at which point another diner will leave the table to try that dish and something else. And so it goes at a buffet restaurant, hunting and gathering with too many temptations and no table service.

Fried Chicken and Steak

What you should be looking for are places where you and your relative or friend with diabetes can get low-fat, low-cholesterol dishes with generous portions of fruits and vegetables. Two eateries where you're not likely to find these choices in abundance are in fried chicken restaurants and steakhouses that advertise extra-large portions. In fact, the beef served in most restaurants is USDA Prime—the highest in fat and calories. If there's no alternative to ordering beef, at least have a very small portion (doggie-bag the rest), and order it well done so that some of the fat drips off.

You know that fried chicken is high in fat. There is a crispy version that is even fattier. One regular breast is 276 calories with 17 grams of fat. The extra-crispy version has 350 calories and 21 grams of fat. The side dishes that are traditionally served with fried chicken are better avoided too. That includes the coleslaw, fries, sugary baked beans, and onion rings. The best choices as far as low fat goes are corn on the cob and mashed potatoes without gravy.[3]

Again, you do not control the voice of your friend or relative with diabetes and he or she may order the dreaded crispy chicken. You will have to just bite your tongue when "You shouldn't have that!" threatens to escape from your lips. What you can do, however, is mention, in a low-key way, that you just learned that the extra-crispy chicken has more fat than the regular kind. Try being amazed and glad you found out and offer this valuable nutrition fact to your friend or relative as a gift, not a condemnation.

Vegetarian

Vegetarian restaurants can be healthy or not. It depends on whether they go heavy on cream sauces, cheese, and nuts to make up for the meat they leave out. They also frequently serve huge muffins, which they bill as healthy because they are made from whole grains and without sugar, though they are frequently full of fat and honey (or some other so-called "natural" sweetener). The sweeteners that cane and beets produce are just as natural as the sweetener bees produce, and all three raise blood sugar. "Natural" does not mean "healthy." Remember that lard is 100 percent "natural," but no one is recommending that you make it a staple of your diet.

Seafood

Seafood restaurants usually have a good variety of low-fat protein. Try to avoid anything fried, breaded, dipped in batter, or served in a creamy sauce, such as lobster Newburg or thermidor. Tartar sauce and mayonnaise-based dill sauces should be used sparingly, while lemon juice can be used lavishly.

Good cooking methods to choose from are barbecued, grilled, roasted, steamed, or stir-fried. (Cajun blackened fish is usually fried).

---

[3] Both corn on the cob and mashed potatoes are considered starch/bread foods so someone who is counting exchanges or grams of carbohydrate will monitor portion sizes with these foods.

French

French restaurants may offer both high-fat choices and healthier dishes. It depends largely on the specialty of the house.

French restaurants that specialize in food from the north of France tend toward dishes with organ meats, paté, goose, sausage, lard, creamy sauces, quiche, and croissants. These are high in fat and cholesterol.

Restaurants with food based on southern France's cuisine are more likely to use seafood, vegetables, wine, and small amounts of olive oil. Bouillabaisse, coq au vin, and salade Niçoise[4] would be good choices.

Even if you can't find a southern French restaurant, though, you may be able to get food prepared as you and your friend or family member with diabetes prefer and stay within your fat budget. The staff in a French or continental restaurant seem to be more accustomed to fussy eaters, so requests to serve the sauce on the side or to cook without butter are accepted with aplomb. Also, the portion sizes are usually not so large as to lead one into overeating.

One caution—pastry carts are very tempting. It's best not to let one be brought to your table. ("An ounce of prevention . . ..")

Italian

Like French cuisine, Italian food varies greatly by region. The northern provinces tend to use more cream and meat. The southern areas, especially Sicily, go heavier on spicy tomato sauce.

In general, avoid pasta in butter, cheese, oil, cream, pancetta, or pesto sauce. Also avoid sausage, salami, cheese, and bread drenched in oil or butter (garlic bread).

Good choices are tomato-based pasta sauces such as marinara, light red, vegetable, and red seafood. Order veal piccata, chicken cacciatore, shrimp scampi sautéed in wine, or pizza with vegetable toppings, double the tomato sauce, and half the cheese.

By avoiding the rich foods and mentioning your healthier eating goals, you may inspire and give added weight to what your dining partner has surely heard before but may have thought was "too hard" for "regular people."

You can even get your diabetic dining partner in the mood for the healthier choices by raving about them when you propose the restaurant. Say something like, "Let's go to Roma's Ristorante. I hear it's romantic and they have a marvelous chicken cacciatore. And I know how much you like chicken."

---

[4] This salad has olives and hardboiled eggs but leaving the yolks and most of the olives on your plate, makes this a low fat, low cholesterol choice.

Making Sense of The Menu

This brings us to the issue of how to find out exactly what is in the "pasta primavera" or the "trout almondine" and how to get it modified.

Ask Questions

You or your diabetic family member or friend must ask the waiter or waitress questions. Pasta primavera may *sound* healthy, but if those noodles and vegetables are bound together with a cheese, cream, and butter sauce, it's a high calorie artery-clogger. You need to learn what's in "mystery" dishes. If the order taker doesn't know, expect him or her to disappear into the kitchen and find out. Don't settle for "I *think* that's made with skim milk" or "That dish probably has pineapple juice, not corn syrup." Beware, also, of the "yes" person who just wants you to finish ordering and will say anything to speed up the process.

This is a great time for you to take the active role as questioner. If you ask for your own knowledge, your friend will not be made to feel different, and you will both get the information.

Request Substitutions

Not only do you sometimes need to know what's in a dish and how it's prepared, you may want to make substitutions. But what if your friend or family member with diabetes is shy, and before the waiter came to take the order, he or she said, "It's too bad that comes with French fries, I'm trying to cut down on fried foods." You know she'd like to skip the potatoes, so you, as the bolder one, can do the asking for her. This can be done in a way that does not single her out as different. For example, you can ask, "Can the fish be grilled without butter and served with lemon instead of the almond butter sauce?" Or, "Could tomato slices be substituted for the French fries that come with that dish?" Or, "Can that be made with an egg substitute?"

Getting food cooked differently or ordering items on the side is much easier than it used to be. Even the fast food chains will make it "your way," an accommodation which was unheard of not long ago.

Making Good Menu Choices

Here are some ordering tips to cut down on temptation and set a great example for your dining partner with diabetes:

1. Ask for a doggy bag when the food is served and "bag" whatever is not a sane portion *before* you start eating.

2. If doggy-bagging is not an elegant option (such as at a banquet), sprinkle gobs of pepper on the forbidden food or portion, to render it inedible and free you from later pangs of temptation.

3. Forget the usual appetizer, entrée, soup, salad, and dessert combination. Try a shrimp cocktail with a baked potato (sour cream and butter on the side), or salad and dessert, or half a melon and soup. This way you won't be eating a lot of food that just happens to come with that entrée and that you figure you've paid for, so you eat it. The à la carte/side dish method is also usually cheaper than the full dinner plus extras.

4. Beware of menus that try to direct you to a safe choice. Often there is an infamous "Dieters's Special" that consists of a 6 to 8-ounce fried hamburger patty with a scoop of high-fat (creamed) cottage cheese accompanied by canned fruit in heavy syrup. It has about 700 calories and more than 40 grams of fat.
    The much healthier "dieter's special" that I would recommend is a turkey breast sandwich on whole wheat or sourdough bread, with the mayo on the side. Almost anything is better than chips or fries, but the best substitutes would be tomato slices or a green salad with low-cal dressing, lemon juice, or vinegar.

5. Pass up foods that are described using any of these words:

Almondine	Escaloped	Salad (if it means
Au fromage	Fried	mayonnaise is an
Au gratin	Gravy	ingredient, as in
Au lait	Hollandaise	tuna, chicken,
Basted	In cheese sauce	macaroni salad,
Breaded	In its own gravy	cole slaw, etc.)
Buttered	Marinated	Sauce
Creamed/creamy	Pan-fried	Sautéed
Crispy		Stuffed

6. Try to choose dishes that are described by these words:

Baked	Grilled	Roasted	Steamed
Boiled	Lean	Skinless	Stir-fried
Broiled			

7. Condiments loaded with fats or sugar include:

Cranberry sauce	Salad dressing	Tartar sauce
Mayonnaise	Sour cream	Teriyaki sauce

You should be able to shock and amaze your audience by telling them that salad dressing (except for low-fat versions) has more calories than hot fudge sauce, ladle for ladle. You could even add that you read that if diet dressing is not available, the next best choice is a small portion of a runny dressing, since most of that ends up at the bottom of the salad bowl.

Another option is to have the dressing on the side, dip your fork into the dressing, and then stab some salad with the anointed fork. No chance of getting too much dressing that way but every bite will have some.

8. Instead of mayonnaise, tartar sauce, and oily salad dressings, use condiments such as:

Chili peppers	Lemon juice	Soy sauce
Cocktail sauce*	Mustard	Tabasco sauce
Horseradish	Pickles	Taco sauce*
Ketchup*	Salsa	Vinegar
		Worcestershire sauce

* These have some sugar and should be limited to a total of 2 to 3 tablespoons a day to still be considered a "free food."

9. Carry your own favorite diet salad dressing, thereby encouraging your friend to bring dietetic condiments, diet maple syrup, jelly, chilies, or whatever will make staying within your goals more palatable. Individual packets of diabetic products are available at diabetes supply stores and by mail order.[5]

My husband carries his own artificial sweetener because he prefers it to the brand usually available. In truth, we often carry a lot more than

---

[5] See Resources in the appendix for mail order companies. Check your phone book under *Diabetes* for local stores that carry diabetes supplies.

that. If we know there will not be a low-fat salad dressing, we bring our own. If he plans on ordering a particular sandwich, he brings his hot chili peppers. His instant coffee is less strong than restaurant coffee, so he brings that too, asks and pays for tea, gives the tea bag to me, and just uses the pot of hot water. It's not difficult to have the best of both worlds— the variety and service of dining out *with* the comforts of home.

10.   Soup is a great way to start a meal. Studies have shown that the calories in soup (not *cream* of anything, though) are a bargain because we tend to eat less of the rest of the meal.

Other good appetizers are fresh vegetables and salsa, seafood cocktail, marinated vegetables, and seviche. Ones to avoid include nachos, guacamole, deep-fried mozzarella sticks, egg rolls, and buffalo wings.

If no one else will order the seviche or marinated vegetables, be the adventurous one and by sharing, maybe introduce someone else (hopefully you-know-who) to a healthier alternative.

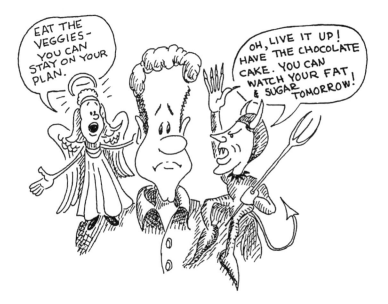

Be Loyal to Restaurants That Listen

Eating at a particular restaurant regularly makes requests for special preparation or substitutions easier and more likely to be honored. Valued customers can usually write their own menu selections *and* get a smile.

Remember that the restaurant wants your business, so whatever you need to take care of yourselves—whether that is information about ingredients and preparation or substitutions—will probably be provided. Sometimes you'll meet an uncooperative server or manager. Fortunately, in my experience, these are the rare exceptions, but they do happen, and it helps to have an alternate selection or even a different restaurant in mind in case you can't get what you need. I've probably encountered half a dozen in many years of restaurant eating.

I once tried to order a pizza with double tomato sauce and no cheese. The proprietor said that was too complicated for her cook to prepare. I left. It was easy to leave because I was with my husband, who supports my efforts to control my fat and cholesterol intake. I wonder if I would have left, though, if I'd been with someone that had decided that this pizza place was "it" and had been unsympathetic or reluctant to leave. There are times when being with our friends seems more important than being good to ourselves. Don't force your friends to make that choice.

Your Help Is Valuable

You and John's colleague Susan (from our opening scenario) now know how important meal timing and avoiding alcohol can be to helping John stay safe. You can explain to others that John *has* to eat between 6:00 and 7:00 P.M. not because he's a picky guy, but because his mealtime has to match the insulin he's already taken.

When Susan learns more about diabetes, she can steer the group to eating within John's timetable and can choose a restaurant that offers many choices of foods low in cholesterol, fat, calories, and sugar.

One way to head people toward choosing restaurants with the healthiest foods is to name three restaurants you know serve healthy dishes and let the group choose from among the three.

> People seldom improve when they have no
> other model but themselves to copy after.
>
> Oliver Goldsmith.

Why the emphasis on your choosing more foods that are low in fat, sugar, and salt and high in fiber? (1) For your own better health. (2)

Because if you're only a *coach* and not a *player*, you risk seeming to be a nag. If you *join* the person, you can rejoice together at great "finds," such as sugar-free, nonfat frozen yogurt and excellent 95 percent fat-free salad dressing. And you can sincerely commiserate at the still-need-to-be-improved dietetic foods like fat-free mayonnaise and sugar-free maple syrup. You can kid about what each of you thinks the world needs a whole lot more than a good five-cent cigar. My vote is for a luscious, fat-free, sugar-free chocolate fudge—with nuts!

If you're sharing occasional snippets of information about low-fat eating, be enthusiastic, but don't preach. Your goal is to educate your dining partner(s) about healthy eating and perhaps convert a few other people—*eventually*. Rome was not built in a day, everyone does not have to look like Jane Fonda or Arnold Schwarzenegger or have a cholesterol of 150 next week (but it sure would be nice if we all had a cholesterol of under 200 at our next physicals).

Chapter 13
Exercise

Exercise With Type II Diabetes

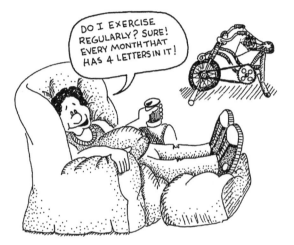

Remember Pat, the fifty-seven year old school teacher with Type II diabetes you met in the introduction? Pat needed to lose weight–at least fifty pounds. She's already lost thirty pounds with a combination of diet and exercise. Her husband was a help with both. Without his joining in her walking, Pat probably would have given up and be on insulin by now.

But she didn't give up because, with his company, walking became a chance for them to get away from the phone and TV and share their day's experiences. They started walking three times a week after dinner and increased that to five or six times a week. When Pat had strengthened her leg muscles and lost a few pounds, she felt more energetic. That exercise bike in the corner of the bedroom that she'd been using as a clothes tree for the last year, looked interesting again. She started riding the bike on rainy days. She even watched some TV while she pedaled away. "It's impossible to rummage in the frig while you are pedaling a bike," Pat says.

So eight months later, Pat had lost weight, had almost normal blood sugar, and had reduced her oral diabetes medication. Her doctor didn't shake his head anymore at every office visit and threaten to start her on insulin.

Needing to lose weight, normalize her blood sugar, and stay off insulin were the reasons Pat got serious about exercise, but they're not why she keeps exercising. Now she walks and rides her bike because she feels more energetic and less stressed. Exercise no longer seemed like work and renewed her belief that she can control her body.

Exercise With Type I Diabetes

For John who has Type I diabetes, planning to go for a bike ride means, just that, planning. He doesn't just call up a buddy, jump on his bike, and ride to their meeting place. He reduces his morning insulin dosage by a couple of units. Then he tests his blood sugar before the ride. His blood sugar at that time tells him if he needs a snack before he starts exercising. For example:

If the bicycling he'll do won't be strenuous (not uphill or very fast) and his blood sugar is less than 100 mg/dl, he has half a sandwich with a glass of milk or a piece of fruit. If his blood sugar is between 100 and 180 he has just a piece of fruit or six saltine crackers. If the test reads 180 to 240, he doesn't eat a snack. For a reading over 240, he doesn't exercise.

It might seem strange that John doesn't exercise when his blood sugar is over 240. He needs to lower that blood sugar and exercise ordinarily does that. However, John doesn't have enough insulin available, if he did, his blood sugar would not have gotten over 240—the excess sugar would have left his blood and gone into the cells. If he goes ahead and exercises anyway, after a few minutes his muscles will send out signals that sugar is needed and his liver will try to help by releasing stored sugar. What will that stored sugar do to his blood sugar level? It will go up even more. Without enough insulin to move the sugar out, it can't be used, so it accumulates.

So even though exercise *usually* lowers blood sugar, it doesn't if the blood sugar is already very high.

Once in a while, when it's over 240, John drinks a lot of water and maybe takes a little insulin. In an hour, he re-tests. If it's below 240, he exercises. What can his friend do while this waiting is going on? He can keep John company and not act disappointed or disgruntled. Perhaps this is the kind of time the sage was talking about when he said, "Stop and smell the roses." Sometime ago, when his blood sugar was over 240, John and his friend relaxed under a tree and talked for an hour. The couple of times this has happened, they still had enough time to take their bike ride.

On days when John's blood sugar is not so high and they start out, his friend can help if John has a low blood sugar. This has never happened when they've only been riding for 45 minutes or so at a moderate pace. But when they are puffing up hills or making a day of it, John can run out of glucose if he doesn't snack every hour. He takes his meter with him and tests from time to time so he knows how much to snack.

If John forgets to snack or underestimates the amount of food he needs, he might get the tiredness, shakiness, sweating, and light-headedness that indicate a low blood sugar. If he knew it was low blood sugar, it would be important to quickly take something with sugar before he feels worse and becomes confused. The problem with these symptoms is that they can be normal responses to exercise that anyone can feel. Blood testing is the best way to differentiate between the two. You can't just rely on the diabetic's assurance that he is fine because when someone has a low blood sugar he often doesn't know it. Confusion may make him unaware of what's going on. Depending on your relationship, and the diabetic's willingness, you might want to learn how to test your relative, friend, or co-worker's blood sugar. The new meters are practically fool-proof and the test takes only a minute or two from start to finish. It's all right to wait for the time it takes to test before giving something to raise the blood sugar. The usual remedy for low blood sugar is one-half cup regular pop or juice. If the diabetic has glucose tabs, give two or three. (See Chapter 8 for more on low blood sugar).

Most low blood sugar events happen long after the exercise is over. From three to thirty hours is the range, although they're most common six to fifteen hours later. Experience helps teach the diabetic what exercise for what duration and at what intensity will lower blood sugar too much. There are steps he or she can take to compensate for that low. A bigger than usual snack at bedtime or a smaller than usual insulin dose are often recommended.

Despite the added inconveniences that exercise brings, there are so many advantages, that it's worth every extra finger stick.

Benefits of Exercise

Can you name three reasons why exercise is good for everybody, including you?

Did you say, "It's good for the heart, helps one lose weight, and builds muscles?" Those are excellent reasons, but did you know there were at least ten? Here they are:

1. Exercise does strengthen the heart. It does this by forcing the heart to work a bit harder. Exercise operates on the heart muscle just as making an arm muscle work harder, makes it stronger. A stronger heart is

capable of more forceful beats so that when extra work is asked of the heart, it can increase its effort without straining.

2. Being able to produce effort without straining means you'll feel more energetic in your everyday activities. Climbing a flight of stairs or mowing a lawn will be less exhausting.

3. Weight loss is much more effective when diet is combined with exercise than with dieting alone. Exercise increases metabolism (the rate at which we use calories) and the size of muscles. Muscles need more energy than fat tissue, so bigger muscles use more calories to sustain themselves even when they're not being exercised. Nice to imagine them using up calories even while the rest of you is asleep.

4. A better body shape is a bonus even if the scale shows no change. Muscle tissue weighs more than fat so even if weight stays the same, the replacement of fat pounds with muscle pounds, especially those on thighs and around the middle, means a slimmer shape.

5. For diabetics the effect that exercise has on blood fats (cholesterol and triglycerides) is extremely important. Exercise raises HDL (good) cholesterol, while it lowers LDL (bad) cholesterol and triglycerides. These effects lessen the risk for clogged arteries that can lead to stroke and heart attacks.

6. Exercise helps reduce the risk for strokes and heart attacks in another way: by lowering blood pressure. And that's not the only benefit; lower blood pressure lessens risk of damage to eyes and kidneys.

7. Weight bearing exercise even has a positive effect on bones; it is associated with increased bone density and reduced osteoporosis.

8. Exercise, along with fluids and adequate dietary fiber, helps prevent constipation. Older people with weak abdominal and pelvic muscles may benefit the most, but it's good for everybody but the laxative manufacturers.

9. Last but not least for diabetics, exercise increases insulin sensitivity by increasing the number of insulin receptors on the body's cells. Since Type II diabetics have a shortage of these receptors, gaining more can lower insulin requirements. Increased insulin sensitivity is an extended benefit to exercise. There is an immediate plus, too, since the exercised muscle takes glucose from the blood even after the exercise is over. It uses this glucose to replenish its reserve supply.

In someone with slightly to moderately elevated blood sugar, exercise has a proportionately greater blood sugar lowering benefit. Because the higher the blood sugar is (as long as it's no higher than 240), the more exercise will lower it. But for a diabetic starting exercise with blood sugar in the normal range, lowering it further can be a problem. That's why snacks and blood sugar testing are such important parts of safe exercise.

10. Even if you don't have diabetes, exercise can be of great benefit to you. One study showed that men who exercised vigorously five or more times a week experienced a 42 *percent reduction in diabetes* compared with men who exercised less than once a week. Even exercising only once a week was demonstrated to reduced risk of developing diabetes by 23 to 33 percent.

If you are overweight and have a family history of diabetes you can help yourself, while you help your diabetic relative or friend. Walk, swim, dance, whatever . . .

Other Benefits

All these benefits are long-term and some of them even require lab tests to confirm their presence. It's not always easy to stay motivated to do something that's good for you when you can't see any difference. Fortunately, exercise also produces almost immediate and positive effects that can make your diabetic relative or friend's, and your, day and night.

11. Exercise improves sleep patterns, mood, and the ability to deal with stress. And the only side effect is a little sweat and a rosy glow.

Risks of Exercise

As wonderful as exercise is for almost everyone, there are some risks for all of the people some of the time and some of the people all of the time. For example:

1. A cardiovascular or respiratory condition may become evident with exercise. The usual symptom that signals a heart problem is chest pain. However, some people do not feel the pain that signals that the heart is not getting enough blood. Only when they exercise do they have other symptoms such as exceptional weakness and shortness of breath that tell them something is not right. Diabetics are especially prone to this condition called "silent ischemia," because of damage to the nerves of their heart.

A pre-exercise evaluation by a physician should reveal any problems. He or she may recommend a stress test. That means an electrocardiogram (EKG) is taken while the person rides an exercise bike or uses a treadmill. This is much more reliable than an EKG taken while lying down. It shows how the heart reacts to exertion. Another way to assess heart function is by taking a twenty-four hour EKG. A small EKG machine called a Holter monitor is worn while the patient goes about his or her normal activity.

A physical examination before starting an exercise program is a must for anyone with:

    a. Diabetes for more than 10 years;

    b. Multiple cardiovascular disease risk factors (any combination of high blood pressure, overweight, smoking, and diabetes);

    c. A sedentary lifestyle in one who is more than 35 years old

    d. Any known blood vessel disease or nerve damage. People with eye or kidney complications need to avoid exercise that can raise blood pressure and further damage the fragile vessels in these organs. Strenuous weight lifting is an example of a form of exercise that temporarily increases blood pressure.

2. Foot injuries or sores (blisters or worse) can happen to anyone even if he or she doesn't have diabetes. Preventing foot injuries and sores starts with wearing proper footwear. Well-fitting shoes that are s-l-o-w-l-y broken in, are a must. Anyone who is prone to blisters will find two-layer socks (sold in sporting goods stores) a help.

Before putting on socks and after taking them off, a smart diabetic checks his or her feet for sores, red spots, and calluses.

Further, anyone with nerve damage or decreased circulation in their feet and legs, needs to avoid activities that could cause injury. Soccer comes to mind, it's darn hard on shins. Going barefoot is also risky and should be kept to a minimum.

3. Hyperglycemia (high blood sugar) can worsen if blood sugar is more than 240 before exercise. Getting the blood sugar back under control is the safest action. Your diabetic exercise buddy should wait until his or her blood sugar is at or below 240 before exercising.

Despite a green light from the doctor, health problems might still occur during exercise. Here are some of the things to be on the lookout for in your exercise buddy:

a. Difficulty breathing or breathlessness that continues longer than usual. This could indicate a heart problem or other condition.

b. Pain, pressure, or aching in the chest, arm, or jaw. These could be symptoms of a heart attack.

c. Unusually fast, slow, or irregular heart beat. Healthy people sometimes feel as if their heart has missed a beat, followed by one that seems unusually forceful. This feeling is usually nothing to be alarmed about. However, if you and your buddy are checking your pulse rate to keep within a target range (more on this later) and one of you gets an unusually fast, slow or irregular beat, play it safe. Stop exercising and rest while emergency help is called or transportation to a hospital is arranged.

d. A rapid heart rate that continues for five to ten minutes after exercise has stopped is also something to have checked.

e. Joint pain lasting more than two hours is not O.K. (A little muscle soreness is common when first starting an exercise program, but joint pain is not.)

f. Dizziness and fainting may have several causes. These could be signs of low blood sugar. The best way to find out is to test the blood. If it is low (below 60), give food or fluid with sugar. If it isn't low, the symptoms could be signaling a need for fluids. If your buddy has been drinking sufficient water before and during exercise (See "Tips" later in this chapter for guidelines), it could be a heart or circulation problem. Get help.

Problems are Rare

It's true that people with diabetes are at greater risk for heart attacks and that after reading the list of symptoms above, you may feel leery at the thought of exercising with someone with diabetes—thinking they may drop at your feet.

This is not likely to happen. It's even less likely, if your relative, friend, or co-worker has been checked out by a physician before starting the exercise program and at the regular intervals his or her physician recommends.

Remember, lots of things can go wrong while you're driving, but you don't sit at home and miss all that's out there, because there's a chance of an accident.

So here are the nuts and bolts of getting moving and learning to like it—together.

Types of Exercise

Any exercise (unless there is some health condition that makes it inadvisable) is better than no exercise. However, there are some kinds of exercise that are better than others. Aerobic exercise is exercise that uses oxygen ("aero" means oxygen). Aerobic exercise forces the heart and lungs to work hard enough to improve their strength but not so hard that they can't get enough oxygen and fuel to the tissues. Unlike *intense anaerobic* (without oxygen) exercise, the aerobic kind can be done for extended periods without becoming breathless. (An example of an intense anaerobic exercise is racing up a flight of stairs. You quickly get out of breath and exhausted because it demands more oxygen than your heart and lungs can supply. That kind of effort can't continue for more than a few minutes).

Aerobic exercise is continuous and rhythmical. Golfing and window shopping aren't aerobic because they involve too much stopping. To strengthen the heart and lungs, they need to work at at least 65 percent of their maximum capacity for a minimum of twenty minutes at a time.

While anaerobic exercise can strengthen muscles, increase flexibility, and be fun, it doesn't burn as many calories as aerobic exercise, nor does it have the best cardiovascular conditioning (heart and lung strengthening) effects.

Focusing on only one kind of exercise could get boring, so doing a variety is a good idea. Just give more time to aerobic activities. Here's a list of both types:

Aerobic		Anaerobic	
aerobic dancing	jogging	archery	housework
bench stepping	canoeing	baseball	gardening
bike riding	swimming	basketball	tennis
walking briskly	rowing	bowling	volleyball
cross-country skiing	rope-skipping		

Even though some of the activities in the anaerobic column can be done at quite a strenuous level, there is usually a good bit of stopping and going instead of the continuous, rhythmic movements in the aerobic column. Again, that doesn't mean they are useless, they just shouldn't be done to the exclusion of the activities in the first list.

Liking an activity is usually essential to wanting to do it. No program will succeed if the person does not find the activity enjoyable and cannot become reasonably competent.

The characteristics of the individual have a bearing on whether it will be enjoyable and "doable." For example, for the obese and the elderly, swimming is easier on the joints than jogging. Those with retinopathy (a diabetic eye complication) should avoid racquetball or tennis unless protective goggles are worn. Someone with poor circulation should avoid scuba diving because of the changes in atmospheric pressure. Weight lifting has already been mentioned as not recommended for anyone with high blood pressure, kidney or eye disease.

That still leaves room for personal preference. The sky's the limit (though parachuting is not an aerobic activity) but keep in mind that expense and convenience can have an impact on how often the activity will be done. If the gym is too far away, or the facilities are too crowded, or the cost of ski lift tickets are too much of a financial strain, you and your buddy will find more excuses for not going than opportunities for going to the gym or the slopes.

Time for Exercise

One of the recommendations given to people who want to start and stay on an exercise program is to choose a time when it is convenient and apt to be done regularly. For people with diabetes, though, especially those who take diabetes medication, certain times of day are better than others, convenient or not.

Exercise in the morning is most effective in increasing carbohydrate use from meals for the rest of the day. The best effects are felt the first 12 hours after exercise when the muscles are replenishing their energy stores by removing sugar from the blood.

For insulin and oral diabetes medication users, exercise in the later part of the day increases the risk of low blood sugar in the early morning hours while still asleep. That's why after a strenuous workout in the afternoon, John eats a larger snack before he goes to bed.

However, for Type II diabetics who are not on insulin or oral medication, after dinner exercise can be done without danger of having a low blood sugar at three in the morning. It's an excellent way to use up the carbohydrate from that meal (which tends to be larger).

Intensity

When people start to exercise they often want to do a week's work in a day. But exercise at too intense a level means the lungs and heart can't keep up and in a few minutes the person is gasping, "I feel terrible, this can't be good for me."

It isn't. The heart is being strained to work at too high a level. And while a healthy heart can take the extra effort, the unpleasantness of the experience turns off the exerciser.

There's a comfortable range of intensity that gets or keeps a person in shape without over-doing it and a couple of time-tested ways to judge if you and your buddy are working at an effective level.

The most well-known is by taking your pulse. Your heart rate should be between 65 percent and 80 percent of your maximum heart rate.

Taking Your Own Pulse

To take your pulse, place the tips of your index and middle finger on the other hand where the thumb joins the hand. Slide the fingers past the hand and just onto the wrist. Let them rest with slight pressure side by side in the groove between the bone on the outside and the tendon in the wrist. Look at your watch and count the first beat as zero. Stop when ten seconds have passed.

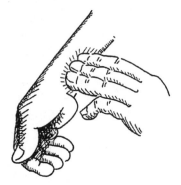

Another place to take your pulse is in your neck about one inch from the center of your throat. Again, use the index finger and the middle finger (don't use your thumb—it has a strong pulse of it's own and you might feel both beats).

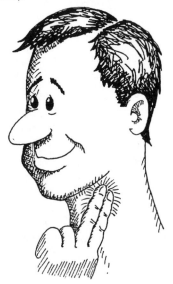

You'll be checking your pulse when you're exercising to determine if you're in your aerobic target range.

Calculating Your Aerobic Target Range

To calculate your effective effort level (target range), subtract your age from 220. That number is your maximum heart rate. You shouldn't exercise at that rate—that's only for running away from tigers.

Once you have the maximum, multiply that number by 0.65 and again by 0.8. Those two numbers are the range your heart should beat in one minute while you're exercising. Here's the formula:

220 minus age = maximum heart rate (beats per minute)
maximum heart rate x 0.65 = lowest effective rate in heart
beats per minute
maximum heart rate x 0.80 = highest effective rate in heart
beats per minute

You really won't find beats per minute a very practical number to use, though. Who wants to count their pulse for a whole minute? Besides, if you stop what you're doing, your pulse slows down fairly quickly so by the end of the minute you won't be getting an accurate rate of what your pulse rate was while you were exercising. So most experts recommend taking your pulse for 10 seconds.

To calculate your range for a 10-second pulse, just divide six into the numbers you got for the 65 percent and 80 percent. For example, say you're 50 years old.

Maximum heart rate: 220 - 50 = 170
Minimum exercise heart rate per minute:
170 x 0.65 = 110 beats/minute
Minimum exercise heart rate per 10 seconds:
Divide 110 by 6 = 18 beats/10 seconds
Maximum exercise heart rate per minute:
170 x 0.8 = 136 beats per minute
Maximum exercise heart rate per 10 seconds:
Divide 136 by 6 = 23 beats/10 seconds

The ideal range per 10 seconds is 18 to 23 beats per 10 seconds for a fifty year old. Remember to go through the calculations for your own age.

There is no point to exercising at a higher rate than this. Some sources recommend not exceeding 75 percent of maximum. That would make the ideal range for a fifty year old, 18 to 21 beats per ten seconds.

Some Calculated Target Heart Rates at
65% and 80% of maximum heart rate

| | Number of Heart Beats in 10 Seconds Level of Intensity | |
Age	65%	80%
20	22	27
25	21	26
30	21	25
35	20	25
40	20	24
45	19	23
50	18	23
55	18	22
60	17	21
65	17	21
70	16	21
75	16	19
80	15	19
85	15	18

Exercise at this intensity level for at least 20 to 30 minutes will burn fat instead of just the carbohydrate stored in the muscles.[1] If your diabetic friend or relative, or you, want to lose weight, exercise at least five days a week. (You may have heard that three days a week is enough exercise to stay healthy. Although it is adequate for maintaining cardiovascular strength, not enough calories are burned to make much of a dent in body fat).

Even if weight loss is a goal, however, more is not better for everyone. The elderly recover more slowly from muscle exertion, so for them forty-five minutes is usually a good maximum time. More than this can result in muscle aches.

---

[1] Ketones are not produced when there is sufficient insulin for glucose to be used simultaneously with fat.

Another Way to Estimate Your Target Zone

Not everyone can use the heart beat formula as a guide. Some people have unusually fast or slow-beating hearts. People who take medication called beta blockers usually have slow heart beats.

For these people there's a subjective method that is remarkably accurate. It only requires that you estimate how hard you're exercising. The method uses the Perceived Exertion Scale.

The range goes from "nothing at all" to "very, very strong." Less than half-way through the scale is "weak, moderate, and somewhat strong." If you have the feeling that you are exercising somewhere *between* "weak" and "somewhat strong," you are working at an effective, sensible level.

Perceived Exertion Scale

Rating	Description
0	Nothing at all
0.5	Very, very weak
1.0	Very weak
2	Weak
3	Moderate
4	Somewhat strong
5	Strong
6	
7	Very strong
8	
9	
10	Very, very strong Maximal

Reprinted with permission, from *Guidelines for Exercise Testing and Prescription*, Figure 4-3, by American College of Sports Medicine, Philadelphia: Lea & Febiger. 1986:23.

If you don't like either one of those methods of determining if you're exercising at the correct intensity, see if you and your exercise buddy or buddies can talk comfortably and still walk or whatever. If you can, you're not exercising at too intense a level. Now, try to sing. If you can all sing, you're going too slow. If you can talk but can't sing, that's perfect.

If your duet makes people throw money, don't stop.

Weight-training: Good for All Ages and Sexes

A recent Tufts University study was conducted with nursing home patients to learn if muscle strengthening through weight training could safely and effectively prevent falls from weak muscles.

In just eight weeks those frail elders increased their muscle strength three to four times. As you might imagine, these were not mountain climbers: they had a myriad of health problems. Some had osteoarthritis (the kind of arthritis most common as we age), osteoporosis,[2] high blood pressure, and heart disease. The oldest weight lifter was 101 years old.

When you hear the words, "weight lifter" does the image of a 400-pound, muscle-bulging man come to mind? It's not that kind of 200-pound barbell-lifting that these senior citizens did.

They lifted hand weights or moved their legs with weights strapped to their ankles. And no one's flannel nightie split from new, bulging arm muscles.

Weight training together with aerobic exercise in a program is a very good combination. Aerobic activities are well-recognized for their cardiovascular effects, cholesterol improvement, fat-burning and other benefits. But muscle strengthening using weights is also a great help in maintaining physical fitness. It even helps with weight loss because more muscle mass means more calories are burned, even at rest. More importantly, it helps prevent loss of calcium from bones which can result in fractures and, as mentioned, fewer falls due to weak muscles.

Weight training requires at least a couple of soup cans (unopened) as hand weights to start. Extend and bend the arm slowly ten times. If that's too easy, if you feel as if you could easily do another ten or twenty, you need heavier weights.

For a full selection of weights, you and your exercise buddy could go to an athletic goods store. Try picking up a weight and extend and bend your arm. When you find a weight with which you can do that exercise only three times, that is your maximum weight for that exercise. If you used a five-pound weight, you need to train with a weight that is 60 percent of that weight, which is a three-pound weight. You should never train at your absolute maximum.

But one pair of weights will probably not be enough. What your biceps can lift, your triceps won't budge. That's another reason why you brought your buddy. Between the two of you, you should be able to buy an adequate selection for every muscle group movement.[3] Some sets are sold as handles with assorted weights that can be switched so you only

---

[2] Brittle, easily broken bones caused by loss of calcium.

[3] Two different hand weights and one set of strap-on weights should get you started.

have to buy one handle. Or there are strap-on weights for ankles or wrists that have little pockets for adding weights so many combinations are possible.

Each exercise should be done slowly 10 times. If you can do more than twelve, add a bit more weight next time. (It won't hurt you to do more than twelve, it's just not an effective use of your exercise time). If ten is too much, stop. You can rest or you can switch to a lighter weight, or do both. This is not like aerobics where continuous movement is necessary for maximum benefit. With weight training you can stop anywhere in the process.

You can learn what movements to make from a video, a TV weight training show, or one of the many books or tapes in the library, video, and book store. Or you can join a gym, or get a personal trainer. I know it sounds very Hollywoodish to have a personal trainer but they are quite affordable, especially if you and your buddy or buddies split the fee. And you won't need a trainer every time you lift weights—just in the beginning when you're learning, and then once in awhile as a refresher or when you want to try new equipment. A personal trainer will be able to tell you how to do each exercise correctly to prevent strains.

Weight training should never be done two days in a row. A day should pass between sessions to allow muscle cells to build new tissue. The nursing home weight-lifters mentioned earlier, did their training three times a week.

If you are a woman, you may be dubious about weight training because you think you'll develop big, unfeminine muscles. That won't happen. You will tone your muscles but not make them noticeably larger. To do that you would have to lift huge barbells as Mr. America does.

Exercise Machines

An exercise machine, like Pat's exercise bike, can be a real plus for an exercise program. Using one can work more parts of your body than your usual activity. For example, if you usually take brisk walks which exercise your lower body, consider a rowing machine or ski-exerciser that gives the upper body a challenge.

Another advantage to having a machine in your home is that it is always available. Pat likes hers because when it's raining or very hot, she can pedal in comfort. I like my exercise bike because I can read the paper, watch TV, and do crossword puzzles, all while I burn lots of calories.

Try before you buy. There are a number of places where you can use the machines before you plunk down a lot of money.

One place is a gym. Considering the price of some machines, it might be well worth a short membership in a gym just to be able to use their equipment and learn what works for you. You'll also get some expert advice from their trainers to help you personalize your choice.

Stores will let you try out their equipment. Plan to use several machines briefly and a machine you're serious about for at least ten minutes at a low effort setting—before you buy. If you know anyone who owns any of the machines you liked best, ask to use theirs for a longer period, two or three times.

There are companies which rent fitness gear. They are listed in the Yellow Pages under "Exercise Equipment."

When you know exactly what you want, you may even be able to get it used at a bargain price through a classified ad in your paper. Try looking under, "Fitness Equipment."

Whichever machine you decide on, it will require real effort in the beginning. It may almost seem like work (ugh). But it won't always be like that. When I first started using my exercise bike, it took a lot of grunting to do one mile. Even after a week or so, getting up to two and then three miles, was almost as bad. But a wonderful thing happened when I could pedal five miles. It stopped being tough and started being automatic. I had evidently developed enough muscle strength in my thighs to make it easy.

The moral is, stick with it, it won't always require the effort it does in the beginning.

Some Words About Exercise Myths

There are some myths about exercise that are more than useless, they can be downright harmful. The first is that old favorite, "No pain, no gain." Exercise done correctly is not supposed to hurt. Even the sore muscles that you may have had whenever you tried some new activity, are not desirable. It's not always possible to avoid overdoing it—sometimes we do our best to go easy only to discover the next day, that it really was a bit too much and that's why the calves of our legs ache.

Another myth is that if you don't exercise, your muscles will turn to fat. Fat is fat and muscle is muscle, neither can become the other. What can happen, though, is that un-exercised muscles will get a bit smaller and the normal fat layer will become thicker if excess calories are eaten.

Myth number three is that the more you sweat, the better your exercise program is. Sweat is water not fat. No matter how much you sweat, your body will only lose water. And that water will need to be replaced by drinking fluids to make up the loss. Rubber exercise suits that make you sweat more, can be harmful. They defeat the purpose of sweating which is to cool off the body by letting the sweat evaporate.

Another common myth is that you can tell how well your exercise program is working by what your scale tells you. Muscle weighs more than fat so you could lose five pounds of fat, feel your waistband get looser, and still not see any change in what the bathroom scale tells you. You lost fat and gained an equal weight in muscle but it will serve you much better. It will burn calories while you're sleeping and muscle takes up less room so you will lose inches.

These myths and old wives tales can sabotage your and your buddy's exercise program. Believing them could make exercise so awful, you'd quit in a week, or so discouraging, you'd quit in a month.

The expert on exercise that your friend, colleague, or relative with diabetes can consult for facts on exercise and diabetes is an exercise physiologist. Your buddy's physician or the local affiliate of the American Diabetes Association should be able to recommend one. An exercise physiologist can evaluate the effect exercise has on your friend or family member's blood sugar and offer personalized advice.

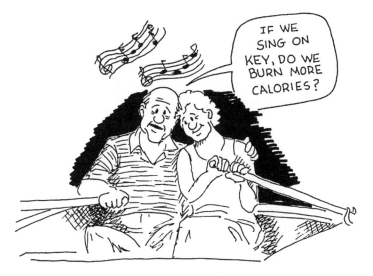

Tips for Making an Exercise Program Work—Together

Imagine that your friend or relative has just left the doctor's office all determined to have a better working body, get off the couch, and start an exercise program.

You know it's important for him or her to succeed, but you also know that turning from a couch potato, into a lean, mean moving machine is a difficult transition. How can you help? Here are some suggestions for maximizing the chances that exercise will become a life long habit.

1. **Do it together.** Together, exercise is a social event not just a chore, though it probably will seem like a chore in the beginning. The time when we as kids, thought running and playing sports was fun, gets replaced by the idea that exercise is a lot like work. Talking and sharing as a twosome or with others can put the pleasure back into moving our bodies. Even as kids we used to play tag and have races in neighborhood groups, didn't we?

Pat found that having her husband's company made all the difference. On the days when she didn't feel like walking, his "Let's go, it's a beautiful day," made her reluctant to disappoint him, so she went. Other times she didn't want him to think she was a slug, so she went. On days he wasn't enthusiastic, she said, "Let's go, I like your company," and he went.

The main reason exercising with someone is better, is that it usually is more enjoyable, and having fun is the most important factor in keeping people exercising. Research studies have shown that while people *start* exercise programs for the health benefits, they *keep* exercising because of factors such as, friendship, encouragement, mental escape, competition and the surroundings.

It would not be a good idea for Pat's husband to suggest a walk saying it would help her blood sugar or waist line. Instead, he and you, would be better served by noticing and commenting that the exercise is pleasurable in itself. This includes not using the daily walk to discuss the family budget, gripes, or anything unpleasant. Use this time as an respite from everyday problems.

2. **Don't try to do too much too soon.** It's the one who is more out of shape that should set the pace. Pushing someone too fast will only make exercise an unpleasant experience and almost guarantee quitting.

Using the heart rate method can be helpful in the beginning. Covert Bailey in *The New Fit or Fat* tells the story of a fifty-three year old woman who said she tried to end a lifetime of taking it easy by running in place. She gave up after five days because every time she ran in place, she'd collapse after four minutes and feel terrible the rest of the day. She hadn't taken her pulse so she didn't know what intensity she'd been trying to work at.

Covert had her run in place for one minute, took her pulse for 10 seconds and found it was 28 instead of somewhere between 18 and 22 which would have been her safe, effective exercise range.

He had her try again just lifting her feet a few inches off the floor. This was still too high and she was soon panting.

Finally, he had her just lift her heels off the floor. That was the amount of effort that kept her in the target range without getting breathless.

This story illustrates how only a little movement in an unfit person can be the ideal starting place.

> *Gear the exercise to the*
> *person, not the other way around.*

3. **Choose a time that you both can regularly devote to exercise.** For co-workers, before or after work may be best. Lunchtime can be great. Take the lunch with you. Eat while you walk (take small bites, though).

Even though morning is best for insulin-dependent diabetics and after dinner is terrific for Type II diabetics who don't take medication, if these times are not great for you and your buddy, do it when you can. Food and insulin can be changed to accommodate your exercise time-especially if it's regularly scheduled at that time and becomes routine.

4. **Carry supplies.** Have fluids, food, change for a phone, and diabetic supplies with you and know what you can do in case of a low blood sugar.

Trained athletes make a point of drinking fluids regularly to replace the water lost through sweat and exhaling. Amateurs, like us, however, think if we're not thirsty, we don't need water. Not so. We can't depend on our sense of thirst to tell us when and how much to drink. This is especially true of older people whose sensation of thirst gradually becomes very unreliable.

Here is the minimum amount of fluid you and your buddy will need when you're exercising. (You will each need even more if it's very hot or you're exercising strenuously).

> 1 cup of water 15 minutes before exercise
> 1/2 cup of water every 15 minutes of exercise
> 1 or more cups of water after exercise

An even more scientific method of learning how much water you need to replace is to weigh yourself before and after exercise. Drink two cups of water for every pound of weight loss.

5. Encourage your relative, friend, or colleague to wear a medical I.D. bracelet (or buy one and give it to him or her). A diabetic emergency could happen when you are not there.

6. Set goals, keep track of progress, and give yourselves rewards for meeting those goals.

The goals could be minutes you spend exercising, blood sugar readings for your buddy, body measurements, or blood pressure.

Goals need to be realistic and attainable. No measurements or weight goals of a twenty year old (unless you are a twenty year old) or perfect blood sugar level goals allowed. No four-minute miles, either. Goals like these would only make you and your buddy feel discouraged instead of uplifted.

Write down your starting numbers and add to your diary regularly. Don't zero in on the occasional sags in progress. Take a good look at what the general trend is toward your goals.

Decide on rewards for attaining your goals and then give them to yourself. I bet the first reward you thought of was food. We do seem to think that way. Cookies are common rewards kids get for good behavior. You don't have to eliminate food as a reward, though. A cup of non-fat, sugar-free frozen yogurt wouldn't be *bad*, but try to think up a reward that you could both enjoy that *doesn't* involve food. Do any of these sound good to you?

1. Massages
2. Book on tape or favorite music
3. A weekend at a favorite resort
4. A new exercise outfit
5. Tickets to a concert
6. _____

7. Start your own exercise tape library. Buy, borrow, or tape videos from your own TV for home exercise and weight training. Buying a professional exercise video tape has one big drawback. After you and your buddy have heard the same advice, or worse, the cute comment of one host to another on a tape over and over, it will sound like fingernails on a blackboard. You can borrow tapes from a video store and even the library, and you probably should before buying one anyway. They come in all levels of difficulty, for different ages, and physical abilities. I prefer to make my own.

Once I've found an TV exercise show I like, I reserve a video tape just for this show. I tape a half-hour segment and put the tape away *without rewinding*. The next time the show is on, I tape another half-hour after the first. Eventually, I have twelve shows on one tape. Even though I may watch it again and again, it takes me a while to get back around to the first one, and by then it doesn't feel too repetitious. And if you're alternating an aerobics show with a weight training show, you get even more variety.

Consider swapping tapes with other exercisers. You'll learn from each other what features are most important, like level of intensity, music, interesting patter, sexy outfits, and so forth.

8. Be open to suggestions from each other on new ways to exercise. Variety is a key to keeping exercise interesting. Doing different activities also means different muscle groups get challenged and over-all fitness is greater than if you only do one thing all the time. This is called cross-training.

Several months ago my husband wistfully mentioned that he'd like to have a canoe or a rowboat. I wasn't very encouraging. The idea of paddling around in a boat did nothing for me. I didn't mind if he got one but I wasn't going to join him.

He still doesn't have his boat, or even look at ads regularly, or even mention it anymore.

How different this scenario would have been if, when he mentioned his boating wish, I had said, "Let's get one, it sounds like fun." He would have felt less constrained about spending the money and time to get a boat because it would have been for *us*. And who knows, I might have loved paddling a canoe or rowing. Together, it would have been more than just exercise.

It's not too late, though. I'm going to start looking in the classified ads myself.

9. Wet, cold or hot weather doesn't mean you have to give up your walk with your buddy. If the closest enclosed mall to your home or work doesn't already open early for walking, ask the management to adopt this policy. One mall near us opens at 6:30 AM. To show our appreciation we wrote the manager a thank you letter and we shop there first.

Do one brisk lap of a floor without stopping and note how long that takes. If it takes ten minutes and your usual walk is one hour, do five more laps. This timing allows you to stop, if you need a bathroom or other essential break, without getting into an argument about how much time you need to still walk. Notice I said, "essential" break. If you're trying to keep your heart rate up for a true aerobic workout, you can't stop frequently.

The time to stop and browse is when you've finished your laps. That's one of the advantages of mall walking. It provides a built-in reward for your good work. You can shop, look, and people watch all you want *after* you've reached your goal.

Final Bits of Advice

Three ways to start your own exercise program:
1. Buy an exercise bike
2. Join a square dancing group
3. Borrow a two year old

Three ways to increase your buddy's exercise level:
1. Start walking together in a mall three times a week
2. Join a swimming club with a two-for-the-price-of- one offer
3. Buy her a puppy right after she gets new carpeting.

Chapter 14
Pregnancy: A Labor of Love

Pregnancy and Type I Diabetes

For most women who have babies, taking care of their pregnancy starts when they know they're pregnant. For twenty-three year old Shauna who'd had Type I diabetes for seven years, giving herself and her baby the best care possible started months before she got pregnant.

Her endocrinologist (diabetes specialist) told her that it was very important to keep her blood sugar normal when the fetus is conceived and for the critical twelve weeks afterward when its organs are being formed. This is the period when high blood sugars can cause serious birth defects, especially of the heart, nervous system, and bones.

During the rest of the pregnancy, Shauna was careful to keep her blood sugars near normal to prevent the fetus from growing too large for the uterus to support. An overly-large baby could have led to a premature labor. Many babies born to diabetic mothers are large, fat babies. That's because they start producing their own insulin at about the 26th week of pregnancy and will process the extra sugar that they receive through the placenta from mom. That excess sugar will be stored as fat so they grow big and fat. Unfortunately, they are not as mature as their sizes indicate.

Fat babies mean more difficult labors and births with all the problems these entail for both the mothers and the babies.

Shauna's baby girl weighed seven and a half pounds. This may not seem like a weight to brag about, but when babies are born to diabetic mothers, a normal birth weight is excellent. We know from the baby's weight that Shauna did a good job of keeping her blood sugar in a normal range, otherwise the baby might have weighed nine or ten pounds or more, and might have had problems.

Very big babies are frequently born prematurely due to their large weight and have breathing difficulties because of their immature lungs. Further, before birth they grow used to lots of sugar from the mother with high blood sugar and produce an over supply of insulin to handle that sugar. Then, after they're born and the mothers' sugar is cut off, their extra insulin makes their own blood sugar drop too low. If the medical team expects this low blood sugar, it can be planned for and the baby can be kept in the hospital for observation and weaning from its dependence on lots of sugar. In a matter of a few days, its insulin production will be normal.

During pregnancy a diabetic expectant mother is more likely to get ketoacidosis (see Chapter 9 on high blood sugar), a kidney infection, or preeclampsia (a complication of pregnancy that causes high blood pressure and seizures). Any of these could require hospitalization. Pregnancy can also contribute to a worsening of kidney and eye disease and advanced coronary artery disease is associated with a higher death rate in pregnant diabetics. These are all risks that can be evaluated and discussed by the future mom and her physician.

Shauna didn't have any of these complications because she was healthy and her doctors were very careful. She checked her blood sugar often (five to ten times a day is not an unusual recommendation), visited her obstetrician every two weeks for the first eight months and then weekly. She had five or six ultrasound tests, weekly tests of the fetus's heart rate after the twenty-eighth week, a glycosylated hemoglobin blood test monthly, an eye test, and three urine tests that required she collect all her urine for twenty-four hours. After the twenty-eighth week she also counted the fetus's movements for thirty to sixty minutes and recorded the time of day at which she felt ten fetal movements. If there had been any decrease in the fetus's activity, she would have called her doctor.

Shauna and most women with diabetes who want a baby, work hard to give it the best possible early start. Ideally, they also have an experienced health-care team to help. The team should include a diabetes specialist, an obstetrician, a pediatrician or neonatologist, a diabetes educator nurse, and a dietitian.

Doctors who don't know how far pregnancy care for diabetics has come in the last fifteen years, still believe and say, "You should adopt; women with diabetes can't have babies." The first obstetrician Shauna saw when she was considering getting pregnant said those very words to her. Now when Shauna plays with four year old Kristen who is healthy and happy, she's glad she looked for a doctor with the most current information.

Gestational Diabetes

Shauna had Type I diabetes long before she had her baby. But there is a kind of diabetes that comes during pregnancy and almost always goes away when the pregnancy is over. That's called "gestational diabetes."

It happens because the hormones produced by the placenta during pregnancy cause resistance to insulin. In two to five percent of pregnant women, their pancreases cannot produce enough extra insulin to meet the additional demand, so their blood sugars go up. Since they produce some insulin, they frequently don't have the symptoms of high blood sugar (thirst, weight loss, etc.) that typically signal Type I diabetes. Their diabetes is more silent, and can go unnoticed if not looked for. In the past, doctors would be alert to a woman's risk if she had already had a baby weighing more than ten pounds. Nowadays, physicians don't wait for an overly large baby, with all the risks that entails, before checking for gestational diabetes. Between the twenty-fourth and twenty-eighth week of pregnancy they routinely test by having the woman drink fifty grams of glucose, wait an hour and then test her blood sugar. A woman who doesn't have gestational diabetes would be able to process that sugar without her blood sugar going up.

Women most at risk for gestational diabetes are obese, over thirty years of age, Hispanic, Black, or Native American, have a family history of diabetes, or have already given birth to a baby over nine pounds.

Fortunately, gestational diabetes develops only in the later stage of pregnancy so at conception and the first three months, blood sugar is not elevated. Birth defects, then, are not a danger associated with gestational diabetes. All the problems associated with an overly large baby are, though.

When a patient has elevated glucose levels and is diagnosed as having gestational diabetes, the first step is to lower the amount of carbohydrates in her diet. This may enable the insulin she produces to handle her food without needing to resort to injected insulin. Since oral blood sugar lowering medications are not approved for use during pregnancy,[1] her only option, if she can't control her blood sugar with diet and exercise, is injected insulin.

Her dietitian will advise that she avoid most sugary foods (even fruit is rationed), and increase protein. She will test her blood sugar *after* every meal. That's opposite from when most people test their blood sugar. The reason for this change is that she needs to know if the amount of carbohydrate in the meal made her blood sugar go above 120. She even tests her urine for ketones because if she eats *too little* carbohydrate, her body will start using fats. Ketones are toxic by-products of burning fat. She may need to increase her carbohydrates and use injected insulin to keep her blood sugar under control. Fortunately, about 80 percent of the time, gestational diabetes can be managed with careful diet alone.

Testing blood sugar, testing urine for ketones, not being able to drink juice or grab a piece of fruit whenever they want, and maybe *still*

---

[1] Harm to the fetus from oral diabetes medication has been demonstrated in animal studies but there are no adequate studies in humans. Women with Type II diabetes who are taking oral diabetes medication should use reliable contraception.

needing insulin shots, are sacrifices that women with gestational diabetes need to make. Still, a normal pregnancy lasts thirty-seven to forty weeks and the gestational diet and treatment usually only start at twenty-four to twenty-eight weeks. Most women will gladly do what's necessary for three months or so. After all, Shauna did it for over a year and felt it was well worth it.

Even though only about 3 percent of the gestational diabetic moms stay diabetic after the baby is born, about 50-60 percent of the women who have it, develop Type II diabetes in the next five to ten years, especially if they are obese.

Women who have had gestational diabetes should expect it to recur with every pregnancy. They should also be checked yearly for diabetes, and try to prevent it as much as possible by exercising and maintaining a normal weight.

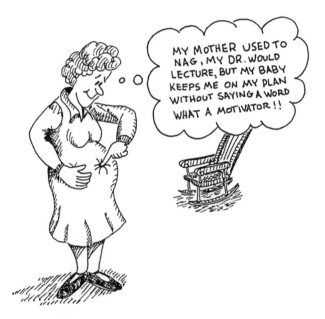

MY MOTHER USED TO NAG, MY DR. WOULD LECTURE, BUT MY BABY KEEPS ME ON MY PLAN WITHOUT SAYING A WORD WHAT A MOTIVATOR!!

Helping A Pregnant Woman With Diabetes

To The Partner

One of the members of the team that a pregnant woman needs besides the doctors and nurse and dietitian, is her partner. Pregnancy for a Type I diabetic should be a carefully planned event with months of preparation to prevent birth defects. Consistent, responsible use of birth control is essential to be sure conception occurs only when the diabetes is under the best control.

The chances of the diabetic mother passing Type I diabetes on to her child are very low, about 0.5 to 2.9 percent. Interestingly, fathers have twice as much chance of passing on diabetes to their children.

A diabetic pregnancy is an expensive pregnancy. Even if everything goes well, lots of medical tests are required. This is one area where if you do have insurance, companies are willing to pay to prevent expensive problems. Compared to paying for extra hospital days, a caesarian delivery, and birth defects, even $4000-5000 for an insulin pump looks like a bargain to an insurance carrier.

Even with insurance a diabetic pregnancy will probably cost significantly more. Couples need to prepare for this so the bills don't spoil what should be a happy event.

To Other People in the Expectant Mom's Life

In the movie *Steel Magnolias* a diabetic woman has a baby she's advised not to have, and dies of a stroke caused by complications of kidney failure. If you saw this movie, do not tell the diabetic mom about it or bring up the concerns that were depicted. This case was not typical of what happens to diabetic women who become pregnant.

If you want to be informed, read anything by Lois Jovanovic, a physician with Type I diabetes who has had two healthy children, takes care of her family, practices medicine, and writes books. You'll be reassured and you'll be able to pass on the good news that with good diabetes control, frequent monitoring of fetus and mother, and team work, the chances of the mother's life being shortened are very slight.

In short, collect *success* stories you can share with your pregnant family member, friend, co-worker. You'll stand out from the crowd.

Chapter 15
Diabetes Is Tougher When You're a Kid

Preschool Children

Of the 123,000 children and teenagers with diabetes in the United States, the vast majority are school age or older. Still, a few get it as infants and toddlers.

Remember how overwhelmed John's mother (Chapter 3) felt when he got it when he was nine? Imagine a mother and father of a six month old who will have to do all the diabetes management of their child without the child being able to tell them how he or she is feeling!

Gloria was a year and two months when her mother became alarmed at her totally sopping diaper and bed, lack of energy, and voracious thirst. The pediatrician checked her all over for a bug but found nothing. He sent her home with reassuring words.

The next morning Gloria's Mom couldn't wake her. A rush drive to the emergency room and many anxious minutes later, the diagnosis was diabetes.

Gloria's mom and dad were devastated. Their perfect little girl wasn't perfect. And "everybody knows" diabetes is passed on in families so one of them was *to blame.*

These are the normal feelings of parents of kids with diabetes and these feelings don't go away easily. They pop up at inopportune times, when parents should discipline but don't, when they should say no to an extravagant request but say yes; the temptation to want to compensate for what they believe is their fault is always lurking. It's not a feeling that serves the parents or the child well.

Gloria got IV fluids and insulin while she was in the hospital and perked up in no time. Meanwhile her mother was given a crash course on what she needed to know about taking care of her daughter—testing her blood for sugar and her urine for ketones, measuring and giving insulin, recognizing and treating a low blood sugar reaction, and much more.

A Parent's Feelings

Gloria's mom felt overwhelmed and terrified. Her dad was sometimes there and listened to the nurse's and dietitian's explanations but he was going to be at work most of the day so it was clear who was going to have to do almost all the diabetes chores.

It is still important for a father or other care giver to learn how to give shots and test blood sugar. Not just for the obvious reason that it gives the other parent a chance to be off duty. The more important reason is so a small child doesn't get the idea that there is a "bad" parent who gives shots and a "good" parent who doesn't.

Meanwhile, Gloria was back to her happy self except, that is, when she had to have a finger pricked for a blood test, or get a shot of insulin. Her mom and dad *hated* to do these things to her but there just was no alternative. Kids almost never get Type II diabetes that can be managed with diet and pills so they need insulin injections and frequent blood sugar testing.

Jet Injectors

For the child who hates the very thought of having a shot, there is a way to take insulin without a needle. Pen-sized jet injectors use a pressurized jet of air to spray insulin under the skin.[1] Insulin is absorbed faster and more predictably than the "pool" that a needle injection produces. Many users get more uniform blood sugar and can even reduce their insulin dosage.

Unfortunately injectors are expensive–they start at about $600 (insurance may cover 80% of the cost). They also require learning how to set the correct air pressure and clean the device.

Managing the Diet

When almost anyone thinks of a diabetic diet, especially in relation to children, "no sweets" comes to mind. But their diet is much more complex than just limiting sugary treats. Milk has lactose (milk sugar), juice has fructose (fruit sugar); bread has carbohydrate that turns to sugar.

Gloria's mom will be saying, "no" to a lot more than lollipops. She'll sometimes have to refuse Gloria's request for another glass of milk or juice or a second piece of toast. It will be a long time before Gloria will understand why her mother won't let her have another pancake—and her mother will dry a lot of tears of frustration that other moms won't.

Low Blood Sugar

Since Gloria can't recognize her own blood sugar lows, her mom needs to test her blood at least three times a day.

There are some warning signs of low blood sugar that Gloria's mother can look for. They are (in general order of appearance):

1. sweatiness	5. stomachache	9. aggressiveness
2. clammy skin	6. irritability	10. sleepiness
3. pale skin	7. crying	11. seizures
4. hunger	8. stubbornness	12. unconsciousness

As you can see, these aren't specific only to children with diabetes. Some are normal behavior for babies, toddlers, and even some grown-ups. Gloria's mom will just have to be a good observer and learn what behaviors *most often* are associated with a low blood sugar test result in her daughter.

Low blood sugar is a real worry for a child as young as Gloria or any children under seven. Their brains are still developing, so a shortage of glucose for their brain cells can cause lasting damage. The goal, then, for preschool children is to let their blood sugars stay higher than normal (this higher range is between 100 and 200) so there will be fewer lows.

Eating and Low Blood Sugar

Do moms have trouble with finicky eaters? Does the sun rise in the east?

Imagine the mom of a baby like Gloria who gave her her insulin shot an hour ago, but has yet to get Gloria to eat the second bite of breakfast. She knows she has to get food into Gloria to balance the insulin but Gloria is not cooperating. Getting tough is not a tactic she can take very often, if ever. Eating can't become a battleground for two strong-willed people. Gloria's mom has to use all her parenting skills to not make eating an issue.

A new insulin (Lispro) has made eating a prescribed amount of food less critical. Lispro acts so quickly, that it can be given *after* the meal in a dosage that matches the amount and type of food already eaten.

Juice (or glucose gel or tablets) instead of candy is usually recommended for kids with low blood sugar. Moms, dads, and doctors don't want kids to learn that bringing on or pretending to have a low blood sugar is a way to get candy. Juice is less wonderful. Gloria's mom keeps little cans and those single-serving boxes of it everywhere—in her purse, in the glove compartment of the car, and in the stroller pocket.

Preventing a low blood sugar is better than fixing it once it happens. Having snacks between meals is one way. Especially important is the larger than usual bedtime snack. It can go a long way to preventing those middle-of-the-night sweaty lows.

Baby-sitters

Another hurdle to get over is baby-sitters. Gloria's mom and dad can't just call up any teenager to sit and then go off to a movie. They have to find someone very responsible, and *train* that person to, at least, recognize and treat low blood sugar. Training means not just a five minute explanation and a pamphlet. It's best done in a couple of sessions along with plenty of, what-would-you-do-if questions. A borrowed video such as "Low Blood Sugar Emergencies In The Diabetic Child" from the American Diabetes Association can be a good teaching tool for a sitter.

When I baby-sat healthy kids as a teen, if they were sleeping, I did homework or watched TV. It didn't occur to me or their mothers to ask me to feel their skin to see if they were sweaty. With kids with diabetes this is frequently done. (At camps for kids with diabetes, counselors make bed check rounds which include putting their hands down the back of kids' pajama tops to feel if they're sweaty). Sweat can mean a low blood sugar. If the child can be awakened, the sitter should give juice. If not, giving a glucagon injection (see Chapter 8 on low blood sugar) or calling 911 is next. Paramedics and hospital personnel can give glucose in a vein to raise blood sugar quickly. Camps have a physician and nurses who can also give glucose injections by vein.

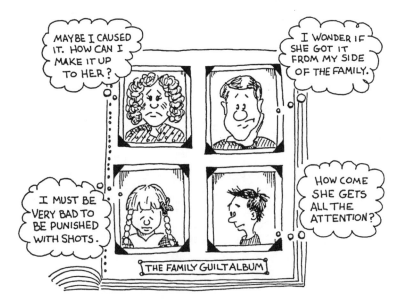

Brothers and Sisters

Gloria doesn't have any brothers or sisters, but if she did that would be another source of problems.

Siblings see the diabetic child getting extra attention and they sometimes become afraid that their own needs won't be met. They feel angry and helpless about this situation they can't control. They also tend to feel guilty because kids under seven or so believe they can *cause* things just by thinking about them and, of course, they must have wished something bad would happen to their brother or sister at least once before the diabetes was discovered.

Diabetes is a family disease. It affects every member. Every member can gain by meeting the challenge of diabetes, from learning responsibility to developing deeper feelings of kinship, and with these, thereby helping to lessen or lose the guilt.

School Age Children

Telling School Personnel What They Need To Know

Half of a school-age child's waking hours are spent in school. Every adult that has contact with the child needs to know what to do if problems, like a low blood sugar, arise. Teachers also need to understand the importance of between meal snacks and, to prevent misunderstandings, it's not a bad idea for classmates to also know why eating during class is permitted for one kid and not for them all.

When nine year old John got diabetes, his mother gave written explanations to John's teacher, principal, and school nurse with precise details about John's diet and treatment needs. In the beginning he didn't want the other kids to know so she respected that. Eventually, he decided it was too "weird" to have his classmates make up reasons why he had to eat in the middle of the morning and why the teacher sometimes gave him crackers after an energetic P.E. class. So John got permission to speak to his class about his diabetes and he, with his mother's help, repeated his "diabetes education program" every year to his new teacher and new classmates. After his presentation, he not only got resented a lot less for his snacking, but his classmates learned how to recognize his occasional low blood sugar events and knew what to do to help him.

Nowadays there are printed diabetes information packets for school personnel (see Suggested Reading), videos and workbooks.

Teachers

John never had a problem with a teacher who didn't want to hear about what might need to be done, because every one was willing to learn and help. But some teachers or coaches are afraid of the responsibility or prefer not to know.

Paula had a teacher who didn't want to hear anything that Paula's mother tried to tell her about recognizing a low blood sugar or what to do if it happened. That teacher just kept saying, "I just can't handle this, it's too much."

Somehow Paula got through the rest of the school year after her diagnosis in October and nothing bad happened.

The next year, she got a teacher who listened intently, asked pertinent questions, and made Paula and her parents feel reassured that the teacher would take care of any problems appropriately.

Kira didn't have a problem with a teacher *after* her diagnosis but her teacher could have been helpful while she was getting sick.

Kira says she couldn't go thirty minutes without needing to go to the bathroom. She was so thirsty that after every bathroom break, she'd get a cup of water and drink it at her desk. At home, her mother didn't know how often she was going to the bathroom because at home you don't raise your hand and ask for permission. You also can pretty much drink as much water as you want without anyone noticing. Kira was a chubby 13-year old, and no one noticed she'd lost weight. Finally, one night she threw up. Her mom called the pediatrician who lived next door, and who, after a few questions, suspected diabetes. He took a sample of Kira's urine to his office and called back to tell Kira's mom to get her to the hospital immediately. Her blood sugar in the emergency room was 510 and she was so dehydrated from her diabetes that her veins had collapsed. It took five hours to get two pumps of IV fluids started and she was in intensive care for two days.

That was nine and a half years ago and Kira is fine but she and her family could have been spared some very scary hours if that teacher had been aware of and reported to her mother her frequent trips to the bathroom and unceasing drinking. No one expects a teacher to know all the symptoms of diabetes or the scores of other diseases kids could have-just to recognize obvious changes and tell a parent about it.

Physical Education and Field Trips

Special school activities can cause problems at first. John and his mother had to learn how to adjust his insulin and food on the days he had P.E.

When John developed diabetes in 1963 there was no way he could test his blood sugar before sports and adjust his food. Today, it's easier to prevent low blood sugar. After the first time that John was excluded from a field trip because a mom didn't want responsibility for what might happen to him, John's mother would call the parent who would be leading the group, explain the facts, and promise to be available at a phone if help or advice was needed.

Blood Sugar Goals

Years ago parents of children under twelve were advised to keep their kids' blood sugar higher than normal. It was assumed that complications only develop after puberty and that normal blood sugar would lead to frequent hypoglycemia in children because they're irresponsible AND physicially active.

Unfortunately, complications can start in children. In one 2-year old whose blood sugar (HA1C test) was four times normal for months at the time of her diagnosis, her eyes already showed diabetic damage.

It's also clear that kids learn and feel better when their blood sugar is normal. Further, hypoglycemia is actually less likely when blood sugar doesn't fluctuale widely. For all these reasons tight control with a goal of 100-180 at least 75% of the time is now increasingly the advice pediatric diabetes specialists give parents.

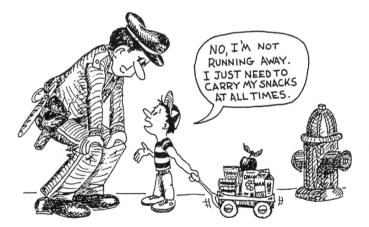

Feelings

School kids need people to listen to their feelings, not so much to get advice, but to really be heard about what's bothering them. And they're not always consistent. Sometimes they like the extra attention diabetes brings, but usually they hate being different.

Remember when John's mother asked if he wanted his classmates to know he had diabetes? At first he said no.

Most kids complain that when they were diagnosed their parents told *everyone*. And they hated that. Some people like teachers have to know but not every mother of every playmate does, unless she will be taking care of the diabetic child.

On the other hand, hiding the diabetes, in fear that other parents won't let the child with diabetes play with their kids, sends the message that diabetes is "dirty" or not nice.

Asking the child who he wants told, in addition to those who must be advised, is the considerate route. Don't forget to explain who must be told and why. And, if appropriate, ask that the information be kept confidential.

Help With Handling Feelings

Children with diabetes know they are different but they shouldn't be made to feel that they are alone. That's why diabetes camps are so valuable.

Support groups are another way to give children with diabetes a chance to exchange frustrations and experiences. In Portland, Oregon for example, there is a support group for parents and children which meets monthly with the children in one room and the parents in another, each with their own program.

Therapists can help both children and parents accept and cope with diabetes. When I asked over 200 people who had had diabetes since they were children or teenagers if they wish they had had a counselor to help them with their feelings, three out of four who had not had a counselor, said they wished they had. The reasons most frequently given for why they or their parents didn't or still don't get this valuable help is: (1) lack of money or insurance coverage for counseling, and (2) not knowing where to find a good counselor.

Teenagers

Hormones do not make diabetes easier. The surge of sex hormones that arrives with puberty usually makes it harder to control blood sugar.

Young women especially, notice that their menstrual cycles change their insulin needs. The increase in hormones two to five days before a period usually requires more insulin to keep blood sugar normal. When the hormone level drops and the menstrual period arrives, insulin has to be reduced to usual or below usual levels.

Teenagers need to be in good diabetes control to concentrate in school and participate in sports. Low blood sugars muddle thinking, while highs cause fatigue. Up until puberty, complications are relatively rare. At puberty, whatever protection childhood (before raging hormones) provides, disappears. Tight control of blood sugar is not only doable, but advisable. The blood sugar range to shoot for after twelve years of age, is 70 to 150.

Unfortunately, many pressures of the teen years work against good control.

Furthering many of those pressures is the thinking that nothing serious can happen to them. Feeling invulnerable is a heck of a feeling for someone with diabetes who *is* vulnerable to short-term complications like high and low blood sugars and long-term complications like kidney disease and blindness. Many teens experiment with drugs, cigarettes, and alcohol. Diabetic teens have all those temptations plus their insulin to "play" with. It's not unusual for some teens to be hospitalized for high blood sugars because they didn't take their insulin. Their answer? "I wanted to see what would happen if I didn't take it" or "I forgot it at home."

One twenty year old admitted to our hospital for the sixth time in two years for ketoacidosis from not taking his insulin, couldn't understand why the nurses and doctors were so concerned. His comment was, "So what if I come into the hospital a lot? My Dad has good insurance."

Feeling different is another problem for teenagers. If you've ever been fifteen, you know what a big deal a pimple was. It loomed and you "knew" that was all anyone was going to see when they looked at you. Imagine being a teen with diabetes and having to wear a Medic Alert bracelet, and test your blood sugar at the pizza parlor, and maybe give yourself a shot, and risk passing out from a low blood sugar if you over-do it at tennis or track?

There are lots of reasons why not wearing the bracelet, not testing, skipping or delaying the insulin and on and on, looks like a good idea at the time.

Dieting

Teen-age girls frequently don't like their bodies at this time so they try dieting. They can get low blood sugars as Kira did (see Chapter 8 on low blood sugar) from skipping a meal. For Kira who was driving, that missed dinner could have had tragic consequences.

People who have diabetes have a way to lose weight that some take advantage of, to their detriment. If they skimp on insulin and let their blood sugar get in the 200's, their kidneys try to normalize their blood sugar by "spilling" sugar. The sugar they lose in their urine is full of calories that won't be used as food or stored as fat. Their bodies will also burn stored fat in an attempt to provide desperately needed fuel. They can lose five pounds in a couple of days without missing a meal. But the high blood sugars make them tired, a little nauseated, and add to their risk for long-term complications later in their lives. It's a bad idea, but too frequently the short term "sure thing" goal of being a little skinnier, seems more desirable than preventing possible complications down the road.

Young men don't usually want to lose weight, they want to build muscle. They hear claims of protein supplements that will "bulk them up" so they buy them. Extra protein isn't necessary to build muscle; exercise and weight-training is. Protein drinks and too much meat and dairy products are a strain on kidneys and add saturated fats that can increase circulatory problems later on.

A healthy amount of meat for a young adult is five ounces a day. That's about two servings, each the size of a deck of cards. Most young men in this country eat three to six times the amount they need. Teenage girls eat, on average, twice the daily protein recommended.

Life Goals

Diabetes can interfere with teens' dreams and independence while growing up, and eventually as adults as well. They may be discriminated against by prospective employers. Some jobs will be out of reach, such as being in the armed forces, being an airline pilot, or being an interstate truck driver (though this prohibition is being reviewed and may eventually be relaxed for insulin-dependent diabetics who can prove they are in good control).

Some of these hurdles (like not being able to join the Army), family, teachers, and friends can do little about. But others, such as helping the teenager like himself or herself more, and make safe decisions are very much within our province.

Feelings

Parents need to stay involved with their teen's diabetes care and not turn over control too soon. It is hard to know when is too soon, what will be seen as support, and what will be deemed nagging. This is important because nagging will lead to anger and resentment.

The best way to show support is to ask how you can help. If you've noticed signs of poor control (more low blood sugar, more crankiness, weight loss, a doctors report of a high glycosylated hemoglobin, and so forth) don't lecture. Instead, try saying, "I'm worried about you. How can I help you manage your diabetes?"

Praise healthy behaviors like testing three or four times a day. Don't harp on the results, which may be high or low. Remember, it is very difficult to manage blood sugar with hormones surging. Every high is not the diabetic's fault. As long as the person is testing, he or she is demonstrating the determination to do a good job—by getting the information that will make it possible to adjust food, exercise, and insulin and stay on track as much as possible.

Unless they tell you, you would only know what their blood sugar was if you looked in their log book or the memory read-out in their meter. Don't do it. Their log book and meter are as private as a diary in which they write about their feelings. If you have a good relationship and are invited to help manage the diabetes, you will know what the problem areas are. If you aren't, finding out behind someone's back will not open up better communication. It might make your son or daughter or friend write down made-up numbers. Even a meter can be fiddled with so that what's in the memory is not the real blood sugar results. It could be control solution. (Control solution is a liquid made by the meter manufacturer with a pre-determined range, either low, normal or high. It's handy for testing to see if the meter is accurate. A normal control solution could be used instead of blood, though, to make it seem as if the blood sugar was normal. Some meters know the difference between blood and control solution but don't count on there not being yet other ways to "fudge" the numbers). There are dozens of tricks kids use to fool adults. Every year counselors from diabetes camps come back amazed at the ingenious scams they hear about from campers.

Camp, incidentally, is not just for pre-teens. Teenagers with diabetes can find it enormously helpful in making them feel less alone. Not every community has enough teenagers with diabetes to have a support group meet once a month. Sometimes, diabetes camp is the *only* place teens with diabetes find peers who understand what they're dealing with. There is only one person in every 600 under twenty years old that has diabetes. Sometimes a teen never has a classmate with diabetes to share feelings with.

Parents can show support by watching blood sugar testing, writing down results, and being willing to talk about diabetes. What teens view as nagging are things like being *reminded* to test. So nagging is out but being willing to take time to be *with* the teen while he or she tests is supportive.

Maybe, though, what one person thinks is nagging, the other thinks of as constructive reminding. One guideline is to consider the first bit of advice a "mention." The second, is a reminder, and anything after that is nagging.

In general, parents tend to turn over total responsibility too soon. Some structure and continued involvement is important even though the young adult *may be intellectually capable* of performing the task.

Also, the kind and level of involvement is different for a fourteen year old than it was only a year or two before. Parents sometimes get stuck in a particular developmental stage and try to continue using the same tactics because they worked in the past. Try new ways of interacting with your teen. Just as Gloria's mother had to find ways of interesting Gloria in eating and couldn't take no for an answer, you too, must not throw up your hands when your teen seems to have "majored in stubborn." Try reverse psychology, try counseling, try writing a contract, try listening—again. Don't give up; his or her eyes, kidneys, feet, in fact, very life, depend on you finding keys to motivation.

Peer Pressure

Parents almost always have a hard time competing with a teenager's peers. What a kid has to do to gain approval from his friends can be anything from merely silly, to stupid, to plain dangerous.

What is the "vaccine" that inoculates kids against risk taking behavior due to peer pressure? It's self-esteem. Teens need to start hearing when they're children, and keep on hearing as they grow older, that their parents love and value them so they will not have to *depend* on their peer group for feelings of worth.

When they are older and usually responsible, they should be told that you know they will use good judgement because they don't have anything to prove to anyone.

Value teenagers for their individuality. They do not want to be thought of as "only diabetics." They are people with talents and "specialness" who just happen to have diabetes.

Chapter 16
Feelings

What It Feels Like to Find Out You Have Diabetes

Being told that your body doesn't work right is like losing something you took for granted.

The first reaction is usually to deny that it's really happening. It's just too frightening to be able to believe.

Celeste, who got Type I diabetes when she was fourteen years old, says she was scared. She didn't want to inject herself, she didn't want any part of diabetes. Her hospital stay helped put diabetes in perspective for her. Here's her story:

> "I didn't want shots; I cried and screamed. There was a girl on my floor who I could also hear screaming and calling out for her parents. I only looked in her room twice. Once when she was screaming. There was some kind of tent over her bed. The second time I looked, the bed was empty and the windows were open with the breeze blowing in on a cold January day. She had had a kidney transplant and died.
>
> "My roommate had cystic fibrosis. The doctors and nurses came into our room often to pound on her back. She was released before me. We corresponded a few times. I asked about her at the clinic, and they told me she had died."
>
> "The third girl I remember used to walk up and down the halls in and out of rooms. She was in a nightgown and pulled an I.V. on wheels. She came in while I was choosing my high school classes for the next year. I told her I had diabetes and they wouldn't discharge me because I wouldn't give myself an injection. I still can picture her face. She couldn't believe that all I had to do was give myself a shot to get out of the hospital. To her it would be like a dream come true. I don't know what ever became of her.
>
> "I was finally discharged even though I wouldn't give myself a shot. They told me that there were 'sick' children who needed the bed. By then, no one needed to explain what they meant.
>
> "My dad had to inject me. I almost didn't let him do it. I remember sitting in the bathroom—my dad with a filled syringe

squatting on the floor with my mom. They were both crying, trying to make me understand that I would die if I didn't take the shots. After a few weeks, I did it on my own. And I got on with my life."

Amanda found out she had diabetes when she was in the fourth grade. She says,

"I was really mad when they told me I had to grow up quicker than my friends. I was so ticked off at the world that I vowed never to talk to God any more. One day I was a chocolate addict and the next I was told NO MORE CANDY. When a dietitian told me about sugar-free candy, I was so happy. That is an invention I love.

"I'm not going to lie and say that I don't cheat every once in a great while. But I don't do it very often because of my fear of AMPUTATIONS. That is something I don't want to have to deal with. It helps me resist temptation."

It's not just kids and teens with Type I that are scared. Bea was 58 when she was diagnosed with Type II. Her father had died of diabetes complications 25 years before, but his was not the only bad diabetes experience she remembers. She came from a diabetic family. Her mother, plus several aunts, uncles and cousins also had diabetes. This is how she felt when the doctor said, "You have diabetes, Bea."

"When I was diagnosed 3 years ago through routine blood work, I went through it all, denial, a *lot* of anger, depression, in fact, I was in therapy for over two years. I could not deal with it, I was so afraid. All I could think about were all the aunts, uncles, cousins, the people I loved sitting in wheel chairs and how active they used to be. Most of them were amputees. And this was going to happen to me? I'm the youngest, 'Why me?'

"After some time went by it came to be 'Why not me?' With the help of my doctor, I set out to learn. I went to diabetes management classes. I learned so much, but it all seemed to be too much, it seemed out of reach. How would I learn all this? Suppose I didn't do it right? So I went back again.

"I joined a local chapter of the American Diabetes Association and that is invaluable. Now I'm Program Director and that keeps you thinking."

Feelings of Denial and Loss

Virginia, was 40 when she was diagnosed with Type II diabetes. It was very hard for her to stop denying that she would have to alter her lifestyle.

"I took oral medication at first and thought that was the miracle 'cure' and I could continue the bad habits that had carried me to the point of finding out that I was diabetic. I went to diabetes education classes . . . actually, I went to one class and went home. I was determined that diabetes wasn't going to run my life. And that included all the brownies, pie, ice cream, monstrous steaks done to a turn, baked potatoes with 'everything,' and veggie souffles laden with butter and cream, that I could eat. Yum! Such blatant arrogance!! The more I ignored my diet, the worse I felt. My legs were numb, my hands tingled, my vision got worse, and my temper flared. My blood sugar rode the proverbial roller coaster. I had yeast infections that wouldn't quit, burning urination, frequent infections (pneumonia, bladder, bronchitis, etc.) and I was always tired. I'd get up at noon, take a diabetes pill, eat, take a nap, get up and eat, and go to bed. What a life!

"One day my doctor wouldn't refill my pills and asked that I come into his office for a blood workup. My sugars had been over 300 for a long time and despite increasing medication to the maximum dose, they wouldn't go down. He broke the news that I would have to go on insulin and I cried all the way home. I was angry. I was angry at the doctor, at my family, at God—I was angry at everyone but myself. This time I went to classes—all the classes.

"I learned a lot in those classes. I learned that being diabetic means I have to take special care of myself. I have to take my insulin or my body won't be able to utilize the energy I give it during the day. I have to eat right, exercise, and take time for myself, something everyone should do regularly.

"I wish I had known years ago what I learned in my class. My mother didn't take control of her diabetes and she died from complications in 1984 at the age of 62. Had I known more about diabetes at the time, perhaps I could have helped her deal with her own condition."

You can hear a lot of the loss that Celeste, Bea, and Virginia felt. They felt they had lost their health, lost the bodies they thought they could trust. They lost their uncomplicated lives that allowed them to eat whatever and whenever they wanted and not worry about high and low blood sugars. Bea, especially, lost peace of mind because she knew what diabetes could do to her—she had seen it ravage her own family. Celeste, Amanda, Bea, and Virginia take very good care of themselves but, still, a little part of them always knows that they are at risk.

Feelings about Food

What would Christmas be without cookies, Easter without chocolate eggs, Fourth of July without ice cream, Halloween without candy, Thanksgiving without stuffing and pie, and birthdays without cake? Celebrations go together with food. In every society food is part of being with people on special occasions. Having to refuse or ration these foods interferes with the sharing of feelings of camaraderie that have traditionally been an important part of these celebrations.

Staying on a diabetic diet means not only rationing the traditional foods that others eat at will, but also dealing with other people's expectations of one's eating. If the diabetic eats the treats, he risks criticism for going off the diet, if he refuses, he may be seen as unfriendly and rigid. A person with diabetes gets to worry both ways.

It's also easy to break the rules of good manners in social eating situations. Some take it as an insult to refuse food, but refuse is what people with diabetes must do. Yet they wind up with "pushers" who insist that, "Just this once won't hurt."

It might be considered rude to ask what the ingredients are before you taste something, but people with diabetes must be wary of hidden sugar and they have to ask and risk incurring the hosts' disapproval. Or worse, perhaps hurting the host's feelings by unintentionally implying that the food may be inappropriate or harmful.

They budget for treats but have to be prepared for the "policeman" who might say, "You shouldn't be eating that." Usually, they say this interference, however well-meant, makes them feel angry.

Feelings About Blood Sugar Testing

Testing their blood sugar is rated as the most dreaded chore diabetics mention when they name things they don't like. They dislike pricking their fingers and testing their blood sugar even more than taking shots. That's not so hard to understand if you've ever done both. First, it hurts more than an insulin shot. Insulin needles are very thin and short (only about 1/2 inch long) and injections are given in places (abdomen, thigh, or arm) that have few nerves, so they frequently are painless. Pricking a finger with a lancet is a different thing entirely. To get a big drop of blood, the point of the lancet has to be thicker than an insulin needle; it's also stuck in a place that has lots of nerve endings. Ouch!

And then there is the pain of the cost of the strips. The money for a days worth of strips could be spent on a lipstick or a sandwich or a day's heat in winter. Nobody likes to spend money on blood glucose test strips so it's not unusual to resent this strain on the budget that most people don't have to endure.

Other reasons also have large emotional components. Some people feel it is a reminder that they have a disease. No one else tests their blood, so doing it makes them feel different.

The results they get can interfere with their activities. A high reading before dinner may mean taking insulin and then not eating for forty-five minutes instead of the usual twenty. Or they may have to delay exercising because the blood sugar reading is too low or too high. It boils down to not being in control of your life.

Every high blood sugar can also seem to bring one a step closer to severe complications and raise fears about the future.

Finally, many people with diabetes feel that either a high or a low is a sign that they did something wrong—like being graded in school. If a diabetic looks at the results this way, there will be a lot of feelings of failure, like getting D's and F's in his or her life. These feelings come up because even the best adherence to diet, exercise, and medication won't give perfect blood sugars.

If waiting for every result is invested with this much negative emotion, blood sugar testing may be avoided as much as possible.

For others, blood sugar testing is actually liberating. It's the key to avoiding embarrassing and potentially dangerous low blood sugars. By testing frequently, they can make adjustments that prevent confusion, passing out, and mood swings that could cause work and people problems. At the other extreme is high blood sugar. It can bring on a sick, sluggish feeling and potential ketones and acidosis.

To people who see blood sugar testing as liberating, results are not seen as rewards or punishments but as clues to action that can be taken. If it's low, the person eats, if it's high but not too high, exercise can lower it. A quick look in the log book can give a clue as to why it went high or low, so whatever it was may be avoided or compensated for next time.

When blood sugar testing is looked at as a useful tool, even the discomfort of sore fingers becomes less important. People who test often say it gets to be like flossing and tooth brushing. You do it because it's good for you and it's just another healthy habit.

Feelings About Injecting Insulin

Injecting insulin is a close second in dreaded chores. It's not so much the injection as what it symbolizes.

When the doctor first tells someone they'll need to inject insulin, it brings back all the horrible feelings of taking shots as a child. Memories of standing in line and hearing other kids cry, feeling doom descend, having someone grip your arm and then hurt you. And those injections did hurt. Long, relatively thick needles were used and a lot of vaccine was pushed into a tiny space (about five to ten times the amount of insulin that is usually injected).

Even when the new diabetic discovers that insulin shots are not as painful as other shots, they still are not pleasant. Learning to stick a needle in one's own body is very anxiety-producing. For the person with a phobia of needles, it is terrifying. I have watched adults cry and cower at the sight of a needle I wanted them to use on themselves. I've been told that for someone with a needle phobia, needing to give oneself shots is like a person with a terror of spiders being told her life depends on letting a big hairy spider crawl on her twice a day. A phobic person is not really sure which is worse!

For Virginia, learning to give herself a shot was almost that bad:

> "In my diabetes classes I met a lot of other people who didn't want to give themselves injections and neither did I. I thought I would rather die first than become a 'human pin cushion.' It took me twenty minutes to muster up enough courage to give myself that first shot. The nurse I was assigned to showed me the proper procedure but my mind (and hand) just didn't want to cooperate. I cried like a little kid; tears of fear and (finally), tears of anger towards myself at having let my diabetes go to the point of insulin. Ignorance isn't bliss."

Taking insulin can also close the doors to some types of employment. The armed forces won't take a diabetic, flying for an airline is out for anyone using insulin or blood sugar lowering pills, and a person who uses insulin can't get a license to drive a truck interstate. It doesn't matter that the insulin user is in excellent control and never has a low blood sugar, it's using insulin that means no federal trucking license.[1] There are enough barriers to the job of one's dream without these additional impediments. Again, there is a feeling of not being in control of one's destiny.

---

[1] The Federal Highway Administration has begun a trial period for waiving the restriction based on a case-by-case medical evaluation. The trial period is expected to start in 1994.

Feelings About Complications

People with diabetes will not want to hear you tell them about your grand-father who had it and lost a foot, or any other diabetes horror story you know. Remember that the threat of complications is always in the back of their minds. In hundreds of questionnaires and conversations, that threat of complications was cited again and again as the hardest to deal with. *Not one person said he or she ever needed reminding.*

People deal with the threat in different ways. Some, like Bea, get on the education band wagon, and learn all they can to prevent them. Between her excellent control of her weight, blood sugar and blood pressure, and the advances in treatment nowadays, the odds are that Bea at 61, will never suffer a serious diabetic complication. But what if her worst fear comes to pass and she needs a foot amputated? Will she feel guilt because it must be her fault? Many do. Everybody goes off their diet once in a while. It may even be a good idea because it makes it easier to stay on it the other 99 percent of the time. But those "treat times" may come back to haunt even someone conscientious like Bea. She could end up blaming herself and feeling guilty for being human.

Some people believe complications are caused by fate. They think that it's how long you have diabetes that makes the difference not *how high* blood sugar was *for how long* that does it. And until recently, many physicians defended this attitude because there was no solid proof to the contrary. Now the Diabetes Complications and Control Trial (DCCT) discussed in Chapter 4 on treatment, has shown us that it's the high blood sugar that is the culprit.

For the people who think complications just happen (I call them *que-sera-sera* people), controlling blood sugar and seeing doctors are a waste of time and money. One eighteen year old young man was admitted to the hospital extremely ill, in kidney failure. He had not seen a doctor in seven years. He had been feeling progressively sicker for months but had done nothing. His insulin had not been adjusted in all that time and, of course, he hadn't had a test of his kidney function. The only happy part of his story is that he had been too sick to leave his parents' home for so long that a kidney dialysis treatment, in a room full of other kidney failure patients, to him was a social occasion—the high point of his day.

But bringing up complications in the belief that they will make some-one with diabetes work harder at controlling their blood sugar isn't a good idea. For years, doctors and diabetes educators tried scare tactics to make patients follow orders. It didn't work very well. Studies show that people are generally so terrified by the horror stories that their brains turn off the rest of the message. They blot it out with, "That won't happen to me, so I can tune out now."

Interestingly, though professionals told patients and families about complications and how to prevent them, they didn't write about how to deal with them if and when they did happen. Until 1993 when Judy Curtis wrote *Living With Diabetes Complications,* no book was devoted to this subject though thousands of people are living and struggling with nerve damage, kidney disease, blindness, impotence, cardiovascular disease, and amputations. The topic was felt to be too depressing.

It is depressing to lose a sense of control of your body, expectations for the future, financial power, energy, and perhaps independence. But it's even more depressing to have your feelings ignored because they're uncomfortable to hear and having limited access to information you need.

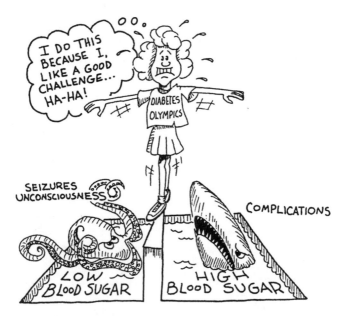

Feelings About Medical Professionals

Hardly a person who has had diabetes for at least five years, doesn't have a story to tell about how a doctor or nurse or some other professional has let him or her down. Carrie tells of many times having to educate an "expert" about the disease. One physician finally told her he didn't have much experience with Type I diabetics, after a year of treating her. He couldn't understand why her blood sugars wouldn't normalize even though she was doing the right things.

Some doctors (and even a few nurses) don't always listen as closely as they should. It's easier to treat a symptom instead of the cause. This happens when several doctors are consulted but they aren't exchanging information.

Sandie told me she went to a clinic where she was seen by several general practitioners and a foot doctor for her swollen ankles and feet. One told her to walk, another told her to prop her feet up, another told her it was heel spurs. Another accused her of not taking her diuretic (water pill) regularly and yet another told her to ignore it, it was just the humidity. When the swelling traveled up her legs and into her thighs she went to the emergency room. As she tried to climb up on the gurney, she collapsed from congestive heart failure due to fluid in her lungs and heart. The last thing the doctor in the emergency room told her before he had her transferred to intensive care was that she should have seen a doctor sooner and taken better care of herself!

Seeing several physicians is a challenge. Trying always to be clear about aches and pains, trying to understand their doctors' responses, dealing with receptionists, paying the bills, and tracking health insurance payments; are endless efforts and very frustrating.

Sandie would approve of Carrie's wish list for what she wants in a physician:

"1. I wish my doctors would consult each other about me, compare notes, make sure treatments and medications don't work against each other.

"2. I wish I could find a diabetes specialist who understood my fears, my desperate need to get my blood sugars under control—and would be willing to work with me daily to see that happen."

In a perfect world doctors would send their patients to the most competent professionals possible, including physicians in relevant specialties, dietitians, exercise physiologists, diabetes nurse educators, and therapists, when necessary. Just as important, though, they would also do these two things: (1) praise their patients' efforts and (2) realize how hard perfect control of blood sugar is.

Feelings About Other People's Helping

Fears about what can happen and the everyday frustration of a high or low blood sugar need to be expressed. Unfortunately, many people with diabetes find their family members and friends don't want to hear it. It's more comfortable for us "bystanders" to have the diabetic be a good sport and not complain or burden us with his or her concerns. What happens, though, when your relative or friend says, "I'm going to the doctor this week and I'm afraid of what the tests will show"? Or, "I get so mad that I have to do all this stuff forever and ever." Do you say, "I'm sure everything will be all right." And "Well, you just have to buckle down and do it, it's necessary."

Chances are, your friend will button up and not say any more. Don't congratulate yourself that his or her silence means you have given comfort. What probably happened was that your friend got the message that the concern he or she had was not legitimate. Now your friend or family member feels more alone and believes he or she'll just have to handle the feelings without help. That's depressing.

It really is hard for someone without diabetes to appreciate all the problems and concerns that someone with it has. That's why support groups for diabetics can fill a void you may not be able to fill. Still, you can listen, really listen. When your friend or relative expresses worry about the tests at the doctor's office, why not say that you can hear how difficult it must be for him or her to wait for results? Ask what it's like. It's not advice or soothing platitudes that are wanted. It's understanding of the concern and fear.

Remarks about the daily drudge of blood testing and shots and diet restrictions are not a signal that you should remind your relative or friend of how necessary they are in preventing complications. Just because he or she gripes about a task doesn't mean that your acknowledgment will be taken as permission to stop doing it. Sometimes, just confirming that the chore really is unpleasant is enough. Consider saying, "You must get very tired of ____. Is there anything I can do to make it easier for you to manage all this?"

One of the least helpful remarks people faced with bad news hear a lot is, "It could be worse." To tell your friend Bob who has just been complaining about the frustrations of diabetes, that he could be paralyzed or disfigured or some other terrible thing and that really what he has is not so bad, is a sure way to make him more depressed. Now he has to feel guilty for not being grateful that he "just" has diabetes. Not a day brightener, no matter how kindly or uplifting the comment might have been meant to be.

Coping styles vary. Some people let news sink in and then forget it. Others worry until they have come to some acceptance or decision. Some worry out loud, still others brood. Accepting your friend's or relative's coping method can smooth the way for mutual understanding.

Men seem to have an especially hard time with a wife's illness or depression. They often feel helpless and inadequate, not feelings men accept easily. So they'll say, "Don't make such a fuss, you're O.K."

If they can't take action and solve a problem they may refuse to accept that there is a problem. A husband might even withdraw and refuse to talk about it. The wife then feels abandoned and angry at him. She may need to stop looking to him for the comfort and understanding she needs and go to a friend or support group. She will also need to stop blaming him for something he can't handle. Counseling may be beneficial for them both.

Good listening consists of the following:

1. Paying close attention to what is really being said.
2. Asking for clarification, sometimes even when you *think* you know what was meant.
3. Reflecting back the other's thoughts with a phrase like, "It must have been..." or "It sounds as if you ..." lets them know you've heard and understood and gives them a chance to explain anything you didn't get quite right.

The biggest mistake people make when they are being asked to listen is to think they need to give advice. That's usually not what's being asked for, but there's a lot of it offered. People with diabetes complain that there's a big difference between advice that's offered by someone who knows enough about diabetes to be helpful, and the usual misinformation. They hear a lot of, "Should you be eating that?" when, yes, they really should be eating that. But what they shouldn't have to do is defend themselves.

I'm amazed at how many diabetics when "attacked" by someone who doesn't understand, take the time to educate. There are a lot of patient people with diabetes who are willing to explain the basics to anyone who truly wants to learn and not just have his or her beliefs confirmed.

Feelings About Being Made a Fuss Over

People with diabetes are like anyone else, sometimes they are willing to be the center of attention and sometimes they aren't. And being the focus of all eyes when the subject is their disease can be even less welcome.

Sometimes it can open up a discussion about health care policy or a genuine request to learn about diabetes. But there are so many times when the stories are about someone's grandpa losing a foot, that people with diabetes become leery of the subject.

Having diabetes is a bit like being divorced. While divorce does not carry the social stigma it used to, it still is not something you want mentioned everywhere and to everyone. It's not relevant in most situations and neither is having diabetes. The one who should have the say-so as to when diabetes gets brought up is the person with diabetes. Having the right to decide is appreciated and ought to be respected.

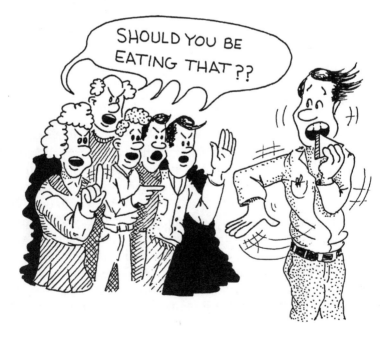

Feelings That Family, Friends, and Co-workers Have About Diabetes

Feeling That You're Doing It All

Family members can get educated, supply the right food, sacrifice for the test strips, medication, and physician fees and find that they are the only ones taking the diabetes seriously. The person with diabetes sometimes makes little or no change. The wife may cook the meals the dietitian recommends but the husband eats cookies and donuts between meals. Or paying for doctor visits and labs fees is a hardship but the diabetic doesn't follow the doctor's advice.

It can be infuriating to do all you can while the person all this sacrifice is for, fails to appreciate it or cooperate. The easy thing is to throw up your hands. The better course is to continue to do your part. It's no different from trying to get a loved one to quit smoking or drinking. It can be a long process to help someone accept that changed habits will pay off.

This is where support groups, subscribing to diabetes magazines, and counselors can be a help. If the person with diabetes is not following the treatment plan because he doesn't think he can, hearing from other people with diabetes that they once felt this way but no longer do, can be a great eye-opener and source of support. Support groups are where he or she can also hear *how* others met the challenge of doing what needed to be done. And the *how* is very important. Most of us think that a person has to believe in the importance of something and when they do, they'll act on that belief. In practice (and many studies back this up), the more we perform a task, the more comfortable we feel doing it, the more likely we are to continue to do it. The belief in it's "rightness" follows performing the behavior. So doing the task even if it seems unnatural at first, is the best way to adopt a new habit. You only have to consider exercise to see how this works. Almost everyone agrees that exercise is healthy but only those who have gotten over the initial period of ineptness or being slow have kept exercising.

If the reason your loved one is not following his or her diabetes program is lack of information or skill—books, magazines, and individual and group diabetes classes can provide the necessary know-how. Classes have a powerful behavior-changing effect because participants are encouraged to practice the skills they'll need everyday. Depending on the class, they may draw up insulin, inject, test blood sugar, write a menu with favorite foods, and so forth. By the end of the class, they can feel comfortable about a task that seemed impossibly difficult before.

If the problem is a more deep-seated phobia or depression, a psychologist or some other counselor should be consulted.

Don't give up until you've tried everything, including sharing your feelings.

When You're Afraid They'll Get Complications

Fear of complications is not felt only by those with diabetes; family members worry about what could happen to their loved one. That's partly what drives them to nag about following the doctor's orders and what makes them believe they have a responsibility to remind and watch and try to control.

Diabetes is more like Hertz commercials than like Greyhound ads. Remember how Greyhound ads said, "Leave the Driving to Us"? Well, Hertz' motto was "Let us put you in the driver's seat." The person with diabetes (after childhood) is in the driver's seat, not Mom or Dad or the doctor; it's just that kind of disease. You can't do it for him or her. If what you're saying isn't working, saying it louder won't work better.

Marjorie was worried about her 19-year old daughter Sandy's overeating and under-testing. She had tried watching every spoonful that Sandy put on her plate. Sandy retaliated by eating "by the book" when her mother was looking and having candy and anything she felt like when her mother wasn't looking. The blood test result numbers in her log book looked great, but the glycosylated hemoglobin test from the lab showed she had frequent high blood sugars. Marjorie had tried scare tactics, got the doctor to lecture Sandy, watched and reminded her and got increasingly frustrated.

Finally, she went to a social worker who specialized in family therapy. The social worker told her that she couldn't change Sandy's behavior, she could only change her own.

Marjorie was afraid to stop the nagging and supervising because she thought less control on her part would mean even worse blood sugars for Sandy and sure complications down the road. In her worst dreams she saw Sandy blind and dependent—on her. This made her feel even worse because she wasn't sure if she was afraid of complications because of what they would mean to Sandy or because of what they would mean to her—Marjorie.

The therapist helped her see these fears as normal and not monstrous. When she was a little more comfortable with her fear, Marjorie changed how she behaved around Sandy. She stopped closely scrutinizing Sandy's plate. She stopped making pointed comments about what Sandy should order in restaurants. She offered to sit with Sandy when she tested her blood but she didn't demand to see the results.

Marjorie's loosening up of control was a relief to Sandy. She could stop using so much energy getting back at her mother and invest it in diabetes care. In truth, she didn't feel very well when her blood sugar was high but she didn't want to do what was necessary to bring it down, because to do that would have been to admit that what her mother wanted was best.

When her control got a little better and her next glycosylated hemoglobin test showed improvement, she was motivated to keep at it.

One day Marjorie told her daughter how frightened she had been and how relieved she was to see her taking better care of herself. Sandy had never really seen her mother's side before. She'd been too busy being angry.

Marjorie did three things right. She stopped being a policewoman but she didn't go to the other extreme and ignore Sandy's diabetes. She still cooked the right food and in a low-key way let Sandy know she wanted to be involved. Lastly, she was honest about her own fear and let Sandy hear, "I feel scared when I see you not taking care of yourself."

Should the Family Change Its Eating Habits?

From the time Sandy was diagnosed with diabetes nine years before, Marjorie had done something else that may have made Sandy's acceptance of her diet more difficult than it needed to be. In their family, nobody else changed the way they ate. Marjorie still bought cookies and sugary cereals and made cakes and pies as usual. For Sandy she bought fruit or products sweetened with saccharine and doled them out in the allotted portions while Sandy's father and brother ate their fill of whatever was the "sweet-of-the-day." It made Sandy alternately sad and mad. It's a common complaint of people with diabetes. They wish they didn't have to watch others eat what they can't.

Sandy's parents reasoned that she would have to see people eating sweets in front of her all her life, so she might as well learn to cope with it at home.

I don't agree. There are lots of things people do to us outside our homes that aren't pleasant. Home should be a better place, a place where people who love you take extra care not to hurt you needlessly. And besides, all that junk wasn't good for Marjorie or her husband and son, either, so why not change everybody's eating habits for the better?

On the other hand, some people who have been raised in homes where sugar was banned, say it became such a forbidden fruit that they went crazy when they were teenagers and could eat sweets at will. I'm advocating a more middle-of-the-road position. Occasional special treats like birthday cakes and chocolate eggs at Easter shouldn't be no-no's to everyone in the family because Sandy can't eat them. Actually, Sandy can and should have a small to moderate portion of these things so that she doesn't feel too deprived. Usually, some trading (she can give up the potato, roll, and fruit at dinner for the cake) is possible so her blood sugar doesn't go too high. This moderate policy makes Sandy less of an outsider in the family celebrations and causes her less resentment. Further, if the everyday cookies and cakes are gradually stopped *to improve the general nutrition of the family, and not because of Sandy*, she won't be the bad guy.

Feelings About Shots and Testing

Friends and family members may find it very hard at first to watch blood testing and insulin injections. Parents may have to do it *to* their child. Not fun.

The really squeamish may wish that these things be done in private. They have the right to speak up. Blood and needles don't have to be out in front of everybody. However, it can be difficult for the person with diabetes in a restaurant, if a dirty sink in a rest room is the only alternative to the table. Consider if it's really something that has to be done away from you or if you can just turn your head away from the testing.

Just the opposite can happen, though. Sometimes a person with diabetes does his own test and several people clamor to have their blood tested too! I've only heard one person complain that testing other people was a problem. I can certainly understand if the expense of the strips is a factor. Once again, the solution is to ask the person with diabetes if he or she minds, and, if you have any reason to think that cost is a problem, find some excuse to compensate by paying for parking or some other diplomatic way of reimbursement.

Feelings About Low Blood Sugar

Taking care of someone who has become irrational because of low blood sugar can be scary. You can see they are getting sweaty and shaky and are confused while they adamantly maintain that they are all right. You know that if the low blood sugar doesn't get corrected, your friend or relative can have a seizure or pass out. At times, help is met with threats or even physical resistance.

One woman told me that she once tried to help get a glass of orange juice into her husband and he threw the juice in her face. That was thirteen years ago and she says she'll never forget what that felt like.

It's shocking to have your best efforts rejected, especially when you get a cold dousing. As long as you aren't in any danger, persist, don't take it personally, and don't leave the person alone. He or she cannot take care of themselves, you are *it*. Usually if you say repeatedly in a loud voice, "Jim, eat this candy," or "Mary, drink this orange juice, you'll feel better," you will rouse the person enough so your words and the sugar will be taken in.

When persistence doesn't work, and you don't have glucagon (See Chapter 8 on low blood sugar), calling paramedics or getting your relative or friend to an emergency room are your next steps.

When the episode is over, again, don't take whatever the person said or did personally. It was a sugar-starved brain that fought or insulted you, not the person you know.

Communication Is a Two-Way Street

Just as the person with diabetes has a right to be heard, the friend or family member does too. I recently read an official report that started out, "Diabetes affects approximately fourteen million individuals in the United States." Wrong. Fourteen million people may have it but many times that number are affected by it.

You have feelings about how your family member, friend, or co-worker's diabetes affects your life and you may need to express those feelings.

Celeste, who has had diabetes for fourteen years, just recently learned how much it had affected one of her sisters. Her sister told Celeste that she was planning to revise her will because her three children weren't in it yet. Her sister then told her that when she wrote out her prior will, she had made Celeste her sole beneficiary because if she ever had any complications, she would need the money.

Celeste confesses that she had a good cry after she hung up. She had never realized how her diabetes affected and truly concerned her family.

Be informed, be kind, be patient, keep your sense of humor intact as best you can, and, most importantly, talk about your feelings and concerns. It's one of the keys to making diabetes manageable.

Chapter 17
Do I Have It? Will I Get It?

Do I Have It?

It's estimated that nearly half of the people with diabetes (about seven million) don't know they have it. They are, almost exclusively, people with Type II diabetes, the kind most often found in older adults. If you had Type I diabetes, you'd probably know it. The symptoms are intrusive, obvious, and, in a matter of days or weeks, cause a person to feel very sick and, without treatment, lapse into a diabetic coma caused by extremely high blood sugar. Here's the list of Type I diabetes symptoms that was given in Chapter 3.

> Increased hunger
> Weight loss
> Tiredness
> Infections
> Increased Thirst
> Increased Urination
> Blurred Vision

The symptoms of Type II diabetes can be the same as those for Type I but they are usually less obvious. Sometimes it's diagnosed on the basis of a routine blood test without diabetes even being suspected. All too frequently, however, a complication of diabetes is diagnosed *before* the diabetes itself. This is what happens to some of the seven million people with undiscovered diabetes. If there are symptoms of Type II diabetes present they usually are:

> Tingling, numbness, or pain in legs or feet
> Slow healing of cuts and sores
> Frequent skin infections or itchy skin
> Tiredness or drowsiness

These are not the kind of symptoms that send one running to the doctor. Sometimes, you're not sure what's significant and what's not. For example, lots of us have aching feet at the end of the day. When is that pain due to more than just normal wear and tear? Or how do you know when a cut is healing slowly enough to need medical attention? And how often do you have to get a skin infection or itchy skin for it to be considered "frequent?" The answers to these questions are not exact but the rule of thumb is, if it's a new symptom or is more severe than usual, get it checked.

Sometimes, the symptoms of Type I diabetes are present in Type II. In that case, you'd probably call your doctor or schedule a checkup without delay. It's the cases that don't have these noticeable symptoms that go undiagnosed.

The bottom line is—be alert for these symptoms and have a checkup just to be sure. Tell your doctor your suspicions, and expect to be given a blood test and perhaps follow-up tests if the first suggests that there is a problem.

If the results are negative for high levels of sugar, congratulations. I hope all your future tests have the same good news.

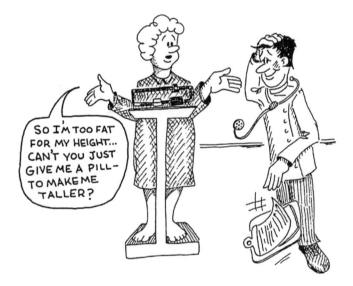

Will I Get It?

You may be worried about your own chances of getting diabetes. Some people are more likely to get it than others. The odds are greater if you:

    Are overweight

    Have had gestational diabetes or have given birth to a baby that weighed more than 10 pounds

    Have a family history of diabetes

Are an African American
Are Hispanic
Are a Native American
Are of Asian descent

Preventing Type II Diabetes

There is only one item on the list above that you can change. You can't do anything about the family you were born into or your ethnic group, but you can do a lot about keeping your weight within normal limits. Moving your body is a great help in making this happen. Exercise does a lot of good things.[1] Exercise burns calories, brightens mood, strengthens the heart, improves insulin use, and increases energy. About the only thing it doesn't do is help you carry a tune!

Muscles that are exercised use insulin better so you're less likely to exhaust your pancreas by needing huge amounts of ineffectively used insulin. Eating smaller meals also reduces demands on the pancreas.

Getting a yearly checkup is another way to prevent Type II diabetes. Yes, I said "prevent." Many people have slowly rising blood sugar for years before it technically becomes diabetes. At the first sign of that increase, portion-size monitoring, reduction in fat and sugar, and exercise (that again!) can push that blood sugar right back down into the normal range. Let that slightly elevated blood sugar be your reason to change your ways. It's not a sure thing, but there's an excellent chance it *will* work, and since exercise and sensible eating are likely to make you feel more energetic and prevent or delay other conditions like heart disease, what have you got to lose?

Pick A Doctor That Speaks Your "Language"

To get the most from that checkup, you need a physician who will help you with your preventive maintenance. But not every doctor will say what you need to hear in the way you need to hear it.

There are two general types of doctors. One is the paternal type who gives orders. He or she may or may not explain why it's important—just that you'd better believe it *is* important and you'd better follow instructions.

The second kind of doctor believes in explaining your test results and your options, and then lets you make up your own mind. The theory

[1] One study of nurses showed that those who exercised vigorously at least once a week reduced their chance of developing non-insulin dependent diabetes by 33%.

with this approach is that if you have taken part in making decisions, you will be more motivated to follow through.

Knowing *What* To Do Is Not
Enough—You Have To Know *How*

Whichever type of doctor suits your personality, before you leave his or her office, make sure you get the tools you need to achieve your goals. These might include a referral to a stop-smoking program, a dietitian for a personalized diet plan, or a session with an exercise physiologist for a safe, realistic exercise plan. A flippant, "Stop smoking and lose 30 pounds," is not enough for most of us.

Preventing Type II Diabetes: a Research Study

Researchers at the National Institute of Diabetes and Digestive and Kidney Diseases, part of the National Institutes of Health are studying people with impaired glucose tolerance (IGT).

If your blood sugar is higher than normal but not high enough to be considered diabetes, you have IGT and are a candidate for this study.

The study's goal is to determine which treatments work best in preventing Type II diabetes. To see if you are eligible, call your local American Diabetes Association or look in the Appendix under Prevention Trials.

Preventing Type I Diabetes: a Research Study

Type I diabetes is believed to be caused by something that triggers an attack by the immune system on the body's own pancreas cells. That something could be one or more viruses, cow's milk, or another environmental substance that hasn't yet been suspected.

A new research study is working on protecting the pancreas cells from attack and death. And since Type I diabetes does have a higher incidence in families with at least one person with Type I, it's those other family members who are being studied and are being offered possible prevention.

Some of the participants are swallowing insulin in a pill form. No, it doesn't lower their blood sugar nor can it help control the diabetes of their family member who already has it. The insulin is too changed by digestive acids to do what it usually does. What researchers think it might do though, is to be absorbed across the intestinal walls and sensitize protective cells nearby which then look for more insulin, finally settling in the pancreas. There they would secrete a substance that may prevent any inflamation and destruction of insulin-producing cells.

Subjects for this study are family members af a person with Type I diabetes whose blood tests show that the immune system attack upon the pancreas has already begun. These folks have a 25% to 50% chance of developing diabetes in the next five years.

So far, over 35,000 people have had blood tests to see if they have the islet cell antibodies (ICAs) which put them at risk. Only about 1,200 have tested positive for ICAs.

If you have a close relative with Type I diabetes, please see the Appendix for details to participate in this important study. You might prevent your own diabetes.

You Can Help With Fund-Raising

Almost all of us can donate some time or money, or both, to increase funding for diabetes research. If you can write a check, that's terrific. If you can't, please donate your time to raise funds or help in some other way. Contact your local chapter of the Juvenile Diabetes Association or your local American Diabetes Association affiliate (they're both listed in your phone book). They will be grateful for your help.

Appendices
Recipes

These recipes are low in fat and have no table (granulated) sugar. While cutting down on fat, especially saturated fat and cholesterol, is important for everyone, even those who don't have diabetes; sugar does not have to be limited by everyone. Even some people with diabetes eat small amounts of sugar and honey.

The advantage of artificial sweeteners like saccharine and Nutrasweet is that their use allows a person with diabetes to have a larger portion than could be eaten of a sugar-sweetened food. Or it means he or she may not have to give up some other carbohydrate source to compensate for the dessert.

Several of these recipes call for small amounts of fructose as an ingredient. Fructose is similar to sugar in that it has the same amount of calories and will raise blood sugar, though somewhat slower. The (slight) advantage is that it is a bit sweeter than sugar so you can use a little less. If you wish to substitute fructose for small amounts of sugar in recipes, here are the equivalents:

> 1 tablespoon sugar = 2 teaspoons fructose
> 1/2 cup sugar = 1/3 cup fructose

If you're cooking for someone with diabetes and you're not sure what he or she eats, you can never go wrong if you ask.

What kind of diabetes your guest has may make a difference in what is avoided. In general, someone with Type I, is more concerned with consistency in amounts of carbohydrates at meals and with limiting sugar, while someone with Type II, who is usually overweight, is cautioned to limit fat and calories–sugar may be of less concern.

Diabetes cookbooks can be bought or borrowed from an American Diabetes Association affiliate or bought in most general bookstores (see Appendix for some suggestions). Your local library may also have a selection of diabetes cookbooks. Choose recently published cookbooks, they will use new products and address the concern for lowering fat in addition to sugar.

Bon appetit!

Broiled Marinated Chicken Breasts

This recipe can be made for the outdoor barbecue or in the broiler.

1 1/2 pounds boneless, skinless chicken breast
Marinade:
2 tablespoons oil
1/2 cup vinegar
1/2 teaspoon salt (optional)
1/2 teaspoon ground black pepper
1/2 onion, diced

Mix marinade in plastic bag and add chicken breasts. Place closed bag in bowl or another plastic bag. Refrigerate at least 2 hours and up to 24 hours turning bag occasionally.

Broil breasts 5 minutes, turn and brush marinade on breasts. Broil another 5 minutes or until only clear, not pink, liquid escapes when meat is cut. Serve with marinade onions. (Makes 8 servings, 3 ounces each)

Nutritional information per serving:
136 calories
25 grams protein
3 grams fat
3 very lean meat exchanges

Chicken and Rice Casserole

An old favorite that's lower in fat but not in taste.

1 chicken bouillon cube
2 1/2 cups boiling water
1 1/3 cup rice
1/2 envelope dry onion soup mix
1 can Campbell's Healthy Request cream of mushroom soup
1/4 cup dry white wine
1 1/2 pounds boneless, skinless chicken breasts
salt, pepper, and paprika

In 1 1/2 quart casserole, dissolve bouillon cube in boiling water. Stir in other ingredients except chicken and seasonings. Season chicken, place on top of rice, cover.

Bake in a 375°F. oven 1 hour 15 minutes or until chicken and rice are tender. (Makes 8 servings).

Nutritional information per serving:
279 calories
30 grams carbohydrate
28 grams protein
4 grams fat
2 bread exchanges
3 very lean meat exchanges

Tom's Kung Pao Chicken or Kung Pao Vegetables

This is a delicious spicy, hot, Szechwan dish that is adjustable in heat. Just reduce the number of chiles to your comfort level.

Marinate together 1 - 24 hrs. (eliminate this step and ingredients for kung pao vegetables)
3 tablespoons white wine
3 tablespoons cornstarch
1/4 teaspoon and 1/8 teaspoon pepper
1 to 1 1/2 pounds chicken breast, cubed

Cooking sauce - mix & set aside

2 cups chicken broth (2 cubes in 2 cups boiling water)
3/4 cup soy sauce
1/4 cup and 2 tablespoons vinegar
1/4 cup and 2 tablespoons white wine
1/4 cup and 2 tablespoons cornstarch
1/4 cup and 2 tablespoons sugar (or 5 pkts Sweet One)

Have ready before beginning any cooking

30 arbol dried chili peppers (in Mexican food section) (Count larger ones as 2 and break in half) (use only 10 for the less brave)
3-5 green onions cut in 1/2" pieces (white and green parts)
1/2 cup canned salted cocktail peanuts (not dry roasted or Spanish)
2 teaspoons minced garlic
2 teaspoons minced ginger root
2 packages defrosted frozen Chinese pea pods (or equivalent amount fresh)

1 can sliced water chestnuts

If making kung pao vegetables, add 1 pkg (1 lb) frozen oriental style vegetables (defrosted) or a mixture of green beans, mushrooms, broccoli, and onions.

Heat Dutch oven or wok with 1 tablespoon oil. Add chili peppers, cook stirring constantly 20 seconds, stir in peanuts and cook together until chilis begin to darken (under-cooking is better than overcooking). Remove from pot and set aside.

Heat another tablespoon oil in pot and add ginger and garlic. Stir quickly.

For chicken version: add chicken. Cook chicken, stirring frequently until opaque (about 3-5 minutes).

For vegetable version: add vegetables after ginger and garlic are hot.

Add onions, water chestnuts, and pea pods, stirring between each. Add cooking sauce and stir. Add peanuts and chili peppers and stir.

Cook, stirring until thickened (about 5 minutes).

Reheat in pot (peanuts do not microwave well)

(Makes 8 servings)

Nutritional information per serving of chicken version:

280 calories

11 grams carbohydrate

30 grams protein

10 grams fat

4 lean meat exchanges

2 vegetable exchanges

Nutritional information per serving of kung pao vegetables:

167 calories

16 grams carbohydrate

4 grams protein

7 grams fat

1 bread exchange

1 vegetable exchange

1 1/2 fat exchanges

Fat-free Oven "Fried" Potatoes

Cutting down on fat doesn't mean giving up potato chips and French fries.

4 medium scrubbed russet potatoes (1 pound)

Slice potatoes in 1/8-inch slices (the thinner the slices the more like potato chips, but the more likely they are to stick to the pan). Place in shallow Pam-sprayed baking pans or cookie sheets. If desired, sprinkle salt on each slice (salt doesn't stick well after baking since there's no fat on the potatoes).

Bake in a 475°F. oven until browned. After 15 minutes, turn slices over and start checking frequently since some of the thinner slices will bake faster and may have to be removed before others. (Makes 4 servings).

Nutritional information per serving:
88 calories
20 grams carbohydrate
2 grams protein
1 bread exchange

Spicy Chili Con Carne

To be sure that I get the very lowest amount of fat in the turkey, I don't buy already ground turkey. I buy skinless turkey breast and grind it in the food processor. It takes seconds.

Alternatively, you can buy turkey breast and ask the butcher to grind it for you but you will lose a little turkey that will stay in the grinder and get a little of what was ground before your order. That's still better than some of the prepackaged ground turkey meat that is higher in fat.

This dish is even better the second day!

You can make a meatless version by omitting the meat, using 1 tablespoon of oil to saute the onions, green pepper, and garlic, and increasing the beans to 3 cans.

1 pound ground turkey breast
1 teaspoon minced garlic or 1/2 teaspoon garlic powder
1 large chopped onion (about 1 cup)
1 medium chopped green pepper (about 2/3 cup) (optional)
4 tablespoons chili powder
1 tablespoon vinegar
1/4 teaspoon ground allspice
1/4 teaspoon ground coriander
1 teaspoon ground cumin
2 cubes beef bouillon
1/2 cup water
1 15-ounce can stewed tomatoes, cut up
2 15-ounce cans kidney beans (3 cans if making meatless version)

Cook ground turkey, onion, green pepper, and garlic in heavy dutch oven over medium-high heat. Stir frequently to break up meat. Cook until onion is soft and meat has lost its pink color. Add remaining ingredients. Bring to a boil. Cover and reduce heat. Simmer the chili for 45 minutes, stirring frequently. (Makes 6 servings)

Nutritional information per serving with meat:
272 calories
29 grams carbohydrate
30 grams protein
4 grams fat
2 bread exchanges
3 very lean meat exchanges

Nutritional information per serving without meat:
196 calories
40 grams carbohydrate
12 grams protein
2 1/2 bread exchanges
1 vegetable exchange

Renee's Bean Salad

This delicious, nutritious salad is even better the second & third day. To marinate every last bean, pour it all in a plastic bag, seal the bag, and set it in a bowl in the refrigerator. Turn bag once in awhile.

2 cans cut green beans (drained)
2 cans kidney beans (drained)
1 medium to large onion, thinly sliced
1 green pepper, thinly sliced (optional)
1 1/2 cups vinegar
1/4 cup oil
20 envelopes Equal
3/4 teaspoon salt (optional)

Mix all ingredients in a large bowl. Refrigerate, stirring occasionally. (Makes 16 servings).

Nutritional information per 1/2 cup serving:
53 calories (add 36 calories and 3 grams of fat if you drink the marinade!)
10 grams carbohydrate
3 grams protein
2 vegetable exchanges

Stuffed Cabbage

This dish comes from eastern Europe, made healthier with ground turkey breast instead of the original beef or pork. (See Spicy Chili recipe for how to get the leanest ground turkey).

1 1/2 pounds ground turkey breast
8 ounces ground or finely chopped turkey ham
2 egg whites
1 teaspoon salt
1/2 teaspoon pepper
1 cup cooked rice
2 heads cabbage
2 large jars sauerkraut
8-ounce can tomato sauce, plus
12-ounce can tomato sauce
1 cup water

Bring large pot of water to a boil and let cabbage soften (about 10 minutes—must be able to separate leaves easily without breaking). Remove first cabbage from water and put second in while filling first cabbage leaves.

Separate cabbage leaves. (May be necessary to return cabbage to water halfway down to soften inner leaves).

Mix meats, egg whites. Salt, pepper, and rice together. Place 1 tablespoon of meat and rice mixture on cabbage leaf. Fold over once, then left and right side, and roll up.

Empty one large can sauerkraut in large casserole or roasting pan. Cover sauerkraut layer with filled cabbage rolls. Cover first layer with 1/2 of second can of sauerkraut. Continue making rolls with second cabbage, if necessary, until all of meat mixture is gone.

Cut up remaining cabbage and scatter on top layer of cabbage rolls. Cover all with rest of second jar of sauerkraut.

Mix both cans tomato sauce and water together and pour over all. Add enough water to cover.

Cook 1 1/2 hours covered.

Serve with boiled potatoes.
(Makes 10 servings)

Nutritional information per serving:
228 calories
17 grams carbohydrate
29 grams protein
3 grams fat
1 bread exchange
3 lean meat exchanges
1 vegetable exchange

Hungarian Green Beans

Delicious and easy. Don't hunt high and low for Hungarian paprika, the generic kind works too.

1 tablespoon vegetable oil
1/2 cup chopped onion
1/2 cup chopped celery
1 tablespoon flour
1 cup tomato or V8 juice (spicy hot V8 adds extra pep)
16 ounces frozen green beans (cooked and drained)
1/4 teaspoon sweet Hungarian paprika
1/8 teaspoon garlic powder

Saute onions and celery in oil until onions are soft. Add flour and stir until flour is absorbed. Add juice and stir until slightly thickened and smooth.

Add green beans, paprika, and garlic powder to hot sauce and simmer 2 minutes over moderate heat.
(Makes 8 servings of 1/2 cup).

Nutritional information per serving:
43 calories
6 grams carbohydrate
1 gram protein
2 grams fat
1 vegetable exchange
1/2 fat exchange

Poached Salmon with Dill Sauce

This salmon poaching marinade is just as good with fillets as steaks.

4 salmon steaks (1-inch thick)
1 cup dry white wine
4 cups water
2 tablespoons lemon juice
1 vegetarian vegetable bouillon cube
1 onion, chopped
1 bay leaf

1 tablespoon dried parsley
1 teaspoon salt (optional)
1 sprig fresh dill
1/2 teaspoon black peppercorns

Mix all ingredients except fish in a saucepan and simmer 10 minutes. Cool to room temperature and strain. (Salmon cooks more evenly if started in cooled broth). Put broth in frying pan and add salmon.

Simmer salmon over low heat just until opaque. Remove from heat and let salmon steep in broth 5 minutes. (Makes 8 servings)

Nutritional information per serving:
153 calories
17 grams protein
9 grams fat
2 medium-fat meat exchanges

Dill Sauce

1/2 cup hot water
1 cube chicken bouillon
1 1/2 tablespoons margarine
2 tablespoons flour
1 teaspoon salt (optional)
1/8 teaspoon ground white pepper
1 cup plain nonfat yogurt
1 tablespoon minced fresh dill or 1 teaspoon dried dill weed
1/2 teaspoon sweet white wine
1 teaspoon vinegar
1/2 teaspoon lemon juice

Dissolve bouillon cube in hot water. Meanwhile, melt margarine in medium saucepan. Stir in flour, salt, and pepper and blend until smooth. Gradually add bouillon and water, stirring to blend. Cook over low heat, stirring constantly until thick and smooth. Remove from heat. Stir in yogurt and dill weed. Stir over low heat but do not allow to boil.

Remove from heat. Stir in wine, vinegar, and lemon juice. Chill.

Makes 8 servings of 3 tablespoons each.

Nutritional information per serving:
40 calories
4 grams carbohydrate
2 grams protein
1/2 skim milk exchange

Turkey Meat Loaf

See the chili con carne recipe for how to get the lowest fat ground turkey meat.

1 pound ground turkey breast
1/3 cup spaghetti sauce
1/2 chopped onion
1/4 teaspoon pepper
1/2 teaspoon dry mustard
1/4 cup bread crumbs
1/2 teaspoon garlic salt

Mix and bake in loaf pan at 425°F. until browned.
Can also be formed into patties and cooked in Pam-sprayed frying pan.
(Makes 6 servings)

Nutritional information per serving:
165 calories
5 grams carbohydrate
23 grams protein
3 grams fat
3 lean meat exchanges

Turkey Dinner Fixin's

Thanksgiving and other traditional family get-togethers may be the standard excuse for forgetting healthy eating but they don't have to be. With only a few changes, favorite dishes can be made as usual, supplemented with some tasty, low-fat, low-sugar newcomers.

Here is a suggested menu: *Recipes that are included in this book.

Roast turkey
Dressing (dressing cooked in a covered casserole outside the turkey is much lower in fat — the turkey cooks faster too)
*Cranberry Relish
*Wild rice with mushrooms
*Sweet potatoes
*Gelatin salad
*Pumpkin pie

Cranberry Relish

An uncooked cranberry relish that is delicious and easy.

1 large orange
1 tablespoon grated orange peel
1/4 cup fructose
1 pound fresh cranberries (4 cups)

Grate orange and reserve 1 tablespoon peel. Peel orange and cut into pieces, removing seeds and connecting membranes. Put orange pieces in food processor with fructose and grated peel. Blend well. Add cranberries, a few at a time, until all berries have been blended into a fairly coarse relish.

Refrigerate in a covered jar several days to ripen.

Makes 8 servings of 1/2 cup each.

Nutritional information per serving:
55 calories
14 grams carbohydrate
1 fruit exchange

Wild Rice with Mushrooms

Very impressive for guests but not hard to make.

1 tablespoon margarine
1 cup uncooked wild rice
4 ounces sliced mushrooms (about 1 1/2 cups)

2 green onions thinly sliced (white and green parts)
2 1/4 cups water
1 chicken bouillon cube
1/4 cup dry white wine
1/2 teaspoon salt (optional)
1/4 teaspoon pepper

Melt margarine in skillet. Add wild rice, mushrooms, and onions. Saute over medium heat, stirring frequently, until onions are tender, about 4 minutes.

Stir in water, wine, salt, and pepper. Heat to boiling, stirring occasionally. Reduce heat, cover, and simmer until rice is tender, about 45 minutes. (Makes 8 servings).

Nutritional information per serving:
114 calories
16 grams carbohydrate
8 grams protein
2 grams fat
1 carbohydrate exchange
1/2 lean meat exchange

Sweet Potatoes

Sweet potatoes don't raise blood sugar more than regular potatoes. This is delicious even without the marshmallows.

3 medium sweet potatoes
1 tablespoon margarine
1 1/2 teaspoons cornstarch
1 teaspoon fructose
1/8 teaspoon maple extract
1/2 cup unsweetened apple juice

Cook sweet potatoes in boiling water to cover until almost tender, about 20 minutes. Peel and slice in 1/2-inch slices. Put slices in baking dish.

In a small saucepan dissolve cornstarch, fructose, maple extract, and apple juice in a small saucepan. Cook and stir until smooth and thickened. Spoon glaze over potatoes.

Bake at 375°F. for about 20 minutes. Makes 6 servings.

Nutritional information per serving:
96 calories
18 grams carbohydrate
1 gram protein
2 grams fat
1 bread exchange
1/2 fat exchange

Gelatin salad

This golden salad is a colorful, light addition to dinner.
Other fruits can be used, just choose ones that are in juice instead of syrup.

2 packages sugar-free lemon gelatin
2 cups boiling water
1 (8-ounce) can unsweetened mandarin orange sections
1 (8-ounce) can crushed pineapple in unsweetened juice
1 (4-ounce) can grapefruit sections, unsweetened

Dissolve gelatin in boiling water. Drain fruits, reserving 2 cups juice.
Stir 2 cups juice into gelatin mixture. Chill until of egg white consistency. Fold in well-drained fruit.

Fold into 8-inch square pan and chill until firm.
Cut into squares, serve on lettuce leaf. (Makes 9 servings).

Nutrition information per serving:
79 calories
19 grams carbohydrate
1 1/2 fruit exchanges

Desserts

Don't tell the kids that this very nutritious dessert is made out of a vegetable! This recipe makes the best tasting, smoothest, low-calorie, low-fat pumpkin pie ever. It's cooked on top of the stove and then poured into a baked shell or for an weekday dessert serve it without a crust in individual bowls and save fat and calories.

Top-of-the-Stove Pumpkin Pie Filling

1 16-ounce can pumpkin
1 12-ounce can evaporated skim milk
1 envelope unflavored gelatin
2 tablespoons cornstarch
1 teaspoon ground cinnamon
1/2 teaspoon ground nutmeg
1/4 teaspoon ground ginger
1/4 teaspoon salt
1/2 cup frozen egg product like fat-free Egg Beaters
16 packets Equal
1 baked pie shell (optional)

Combine pumpkin, milk, gelatin, cornstarch, spices, and salt in saucepan. Let stand 5 minutes to soften gelatin. Cook and stir over medium heat until mixture bubbles; continue cooking while stirring another 2 minutes. Remove from heat. Gradually stir 1 cup of the hot mixture into eggs. Add egg mixture to saucepan and stir and cook over medium heat without boiling for 2 minutes. Remove from heat and stir in Equal. Pour into pie crust or individual dishes. Refrigerate. Garnish with whipped topping if desired. (8 servings)

Nutritional information per serving without crust:
64 calories
10 grams carbohydrate
6 grams protein
1/2 skim milk
1 vegetable

Nutritional information* per serving (8/pie) of a homemade crust:
112 calories
10 grams carbohydrate
1 gram protein
8 grams fat
1 bread exchange
1 1/2 fat exchanges

* Homemade, ready-to-eat, and pie crust mixes vary in ingredients. Check nutritional information on individual packages.

About whipped toppings

Estee makes a dry mix that is sweetened with Nutrasweet. But the light version of frozen toppings like Cool Whip are just as low in calories and taste better. A tablespoon has only 8 calories and 1 gram of carbohydrate. A spoonful on pie or pudding is a great addition.

Chocolate/Vanilla Rum Parfaits

Easy, easy, easy but looks and tastes elegant.

1 package sugar-free instant chocolate or chocolate fudge pudding and pie filling mix (chocolate fudge is darker)
1 package sugar-free instant vanilla pudding and pie filling mix
4 cups cold skimmed milk, divided
3 teaspoons rum extract, divided

Make chocolate pudding as package directs using 2 cups milk. Stir in 2 teaspoons rum extract.

Make vanilla pudding as package directs using 2 cups milk. Stir in 1 teaspoon rum extract.

Spoon vanilla pudding into 8 small wine or stemmed glass dessert dishes. Next spoon in chocolate pudding. Top with whipped topping and chocolate curls or maraschino cherry. Chill. (Makes 8 servings).

Nutritional information per serving:
80 calories
13 grams carbohydrate
5 grams protein
1 bread exchange

Chocolate Cherry Almond Pudding

Kids love this combination of flavors.

1 package sugar-free chocolate instant pudding & pie filling mix
2 cups cold skimmed milk
1 1/2 teaspoons cherry extract
1/4 teaspoon almond extract

Mix all ingredients. Pour into 4 small dishes. For children, top with dollop of whipped topping and an animal cracker.

Nutritional information same as previous recipe.

Other Pudding Combinations

Make 1 package chocolate pudding and 1 package vanilla pudding per package instructions. Mix together to make a lighter milk chocolate pudding. Serves 8.

Other flavorings to add to pudding.

1/4 - 3/4 tsp mint extract to chocolate pudding mix
1/4 - 1/2 tsp maple extract to vanilla pudding mix
1 tablespoon no-sugar-added peanut butter to chocolate pudding
   for a peanut butter cup candy taste

Custom-sweetened nonfat yogurt

Usually cheaper than buying little individual containers. And you can make more flavors by changing preserves and extract flavors. Also delicious as a sauce over fresh fruit.

1 quart nonfat plain yogurt
2 tablespoons Nutradiet Red Tart Cherry, Strawberry, or Black-
   berry preserves or other low calorie/low sugar preserves
16 envelopes Equal
1/2 teaspoon almond extract

Mix all ingredients together. Pour into 6 individual dishes.
(Makes 6 servings).

Nutritional information per serving:
74 calories
10 grams carbohydrate
8 grams protein
1 skim milk exchange

Yogurt/Jello/Fruit Parfait

A nice change from plain gelatin with the added bonus of calcium, fruit, and not many calories.

1 quart non-fat plain yogurt
2 tablespoons diet preserves
16 envelopes Equal (or less to taste)
1/2 teaspoon almond extract

2 0.3-ounce packages sugar-free cherry gelatin
2 cups boiling water
2 cups cold water
1 16-ounce can light fruit cocktail, drained

Mix yogurt, preserves, Equal, and extract and refrigerate in mixing bowl. Prepare gelatin according to package directions. Add drained fruit cocktail. Refrigerate, mixing from time to time.

When gelatin mixture is semi-solid, add yogurt mixture and mix. (Makes 10 1-cup servings).

Nutritional information per serving:
63 calories   3 grams protein   0 grams fat
12 grams carbohydrate   1 bread exchange

Individual Cheesecakes (Fat Free!)

I always get compliments on this at parties and potlucks. People never believe these little beauties are fat-free.

8 ounces fat-free cream cheese
  (brick form, not tub)
8 ounces fat-free cottage cheese
3 envelopes Sweet One
  artificial sweetener
2 tablespoons fructose (8 envelopes)
2 egg whites
1/4 cup fat-free sour cream
1/2 teaspoon vanilla extract

Topping*
1/3 cup fat-free sour cream
1 envelope Equal
1/3 cup light cherry pie filling
1 envelope Equal
1/8 tsp almond extract

Blend everything but topping ingredients in food processor until smooth. Pour into lined muffin cups (foil ones, are especially pretty). Put muffin tin in a larger pan with about 3/4 inch water.

Bake in a 350°F. oven for about 30-40 minutes or until knife inserted in center comes out clean. Chill. (Makes 12-15 servings.)

* Topping: Mix sour cream and 1 envelope Equal. Spread on cheesecakes. Combine pie filling, extract and another envelope Equal. Place 1 cherry and a little sauce on each cheesecake.

Nutritional information per serving with topping:
(12 servings) 53 calories   (15 servings) 42 calories
6 grams carbohydrate   5 grams carbohydrate
7.5 grams protein   6 grams protein
1/2 skim milk exchange   1/2 skim milk exchange

Apple Coffee Cake

So delicious and so low in calories for a BIG slice!

Spray 9 x 13 cookie sheet with cooking spray. Preheat oven to 425° F.

1 package (8 oz.) crescent refrigerated dinner rolls	4-5 delicious apples, cubed (3 cups) 1 teaspoon cinnamon
1 box sugar-free vanilla Cook and Serve pudding mix (NOT instant)	1 8-oz pkg fat-free cream cheese (brick form) 1/2 teaspoon cinnamon
1 1/3 cup water	3 envelopes Equal (or other artificial
1 box sugar-free lemon gelatin	sweetener equal to 2 Tbl. sugar)

Press rolls in sprayed cookie sheet and seal perforations. Bake 6-8 min. or until golden brown. Cool on wire rack.

In medium pot combine pudding mix, dry gelatin, water, diced apples and 1 teaspoon cinnamon. Cook over medium heat, stirring constantly, until mixture comes to a boil. Remove from heat. Cool 15 minutes.
While apple mixture cools, combine cream cheese, Equal and 1/2 tsp cinnamon. Spread on cooled crust. Top with apple mixture. Chill.

Nutritional information per slice for 16 servings:
80 calories   3 grams fat
12 grams carbohydrate   3 grams protein   1 bread, 1/2 fat exchange

Noodle Pudding

Not really what you think of as a pudding. This actually cuts into squares. A European classic.

16 ounces medium or wide noodles	16 ounces fat-free cottage cheese
8 ounces fat-free cream cheese product in brick form	1 teaspoon salt (optional) 2 cups skim (nonfat) milk
4 egg whites or egg substitute equal to 3 eggs	1 tablespoon vanilla extract 1 cup raisins
	12 envelopes Sweet One

Boil noodles until barely tender. Drain, then rinse with cold water. Blend other ingredients except raisins in a large bowl. Add noodles and raisins and stir until well blended. Pour into 9 x 13 baking dish sprayed with Pam or equivalent.

Bake at 350°F. for 1 hour or until light brown.

Chill and cut into squares. Refrigerate. (Makes 20 servings)

Nutritional information per serving:
145 calories
25 grams carbohydrate
14 grams protein
1 bread exchange
1 skim milk exchange

Sugar-free Gelatin Squares

These may be cut in squares or with cookie cutters.

4 boxes any flavor sugar-free gelatin
2 1/2 cups water

Add boiling water to gelatin and stir. When gelatin is dissolved pour into an 8 or 9-inch pan and refrigerate until firm. Cut into squares.

This is a fat free food, there's no limit on serving size.

Non-fat Apple Oat Bran Muffins

These are not only *not bad* for you but are *actually healthy*. The oat bran and apples have soluble fiber to lower cholesterol and blood sugar. They keep great in the refrigerator for a week and freeze well, so you can make the double batch following this single-batch recipe.

2 cups (1/2 lb) oat bran cereal (cereal is the kind used to make HOT cereal, it is 100% oat bran)
1/4 cup sugar or sugar substitute (I use 1/4 cup Twin)
1 1/2 teaspoons cinnamon
1 tablespoon baking powder
1/2 cup non-fat milk
6 ounces frozen apple juice concentrate (does not have to be defrosted)
2 egg whites
2 tablespoons corn syrup
2 coarsely grated delicious or other apples (3 if they're small)
1/2 teaspoon salt (optional)

Stir until mixed. Fill paper-lined muffin cups halfway.

Bake at 425° F. for about 15 minutes. Do not overbake. They are done when the tops feel somewhat dry.

Store in closed container in the refrigerator for up to 1 week. May also be frozen.

Makes 24 muffins.

Nutritional information per muffin:

58 calories	0 grams fat
12 grams carbohydrate	2 grams protein

NON-FAT APPLE OAT BRAN MUFFINS

(Double batch — 48 muffins)

These muffins are such healthy and easy-to-serve refreshments for a crowd (take a batch to a diabetes support group or the office), that I've included a doubled recipe that conveniently uses a whole 1-pound box of oat bran cereal and a whole 12-ounce can of apple juice.

1 pound box oat bran cereal (cereal is the kind used to make HOT cereal, it is 100% oat bran)
1/2 cup sugar or sugar substitute (I use 1/2 cup Twin)
1 tablespoon cinnamon
2 tablespoons baking powder
1 cup non-fat milk
12 ounces frozen apple juice concentrate (does not have to be defrosted)
4 egg whites
1/4 cup corn syrup
4 coarsely grated delicious or other apples (6 if they're small)
1 teaspoon salt (optional)

Stir until mixed. Bake in paper-lined muffin cups. Makes 48.
Bake at 425°F. for about 15 minutes. Do not overbake. They are done when the tops feel somewhat dry.

Store in closed container in the refrigerator for up to 1 week. May also be frozen.

Chocolate Treats

Yummy Chocolate Erasers

These look like erasers but they don't taste like them. Besides being one way to get a chocolate fix without adding calories or raising blood sugar, at 5 calories each, you can have a handful and still be O.K.

1 cup cold water	4 envelopes unflavored gelatin
4 envelopes Alba Chocolate Shake	1 1/2 cups water
6-8 envelopes Equal	2 teaspoons imitation chocolate extract

In a small saucepan, sprinkle gelatin over the 1 cup cold water. Let stand about 1 minute until softened. Stir over low heat until gelatin is completely dissolved. Allow to cool while mixing shake mix, 1 1/2 cups water, Equal, and chocolate extract in a blender. Blend 30 seconds at low speed. Add gelatin mixture and process another 30 seconds.

Pour into a 8 or 9-inch square baking dish. Chill until firm, about 2 hours. Cut into 1-inch squares. (Makes 64 squares).

Nutritional information per square:
5 calories	less than 1 gram carbohydrate
less than 1 gram protein	4 or less is a "free" food

25-Calorie Hot Chocolate

There are a lot of sugar-free hot chocolate mixes on the market but there is only one that is also practically fat-free. That is Carnation DIET Hot Cocoa mix. Each serving has only 25 calories, 5 grams of carbohydrate, and 2 grams of protein. It's practically a "free" food! What a great way to get a chocolate fix in the winter.

Sugar-free chocolate popsicles

Fudgsicle and Weight Watchers both make delicious 35-calorie frozen chocolate treats. The perfect chocolate fix in the summertime.

Chocolate "Ice Cream"

Dreyer's Chocolate Sugar-Free Frozen Dietary Dairy Dessert with Nutrasweet has made me stop yearning for chocolate ice cream. Comes in other delicious flavors but I'm biased toward anything chocolate. 80 calories per 1/2 cup serving.

How to Tell if Someone Has Low Blood Sugar

Early Symptoms
Sweating
Nervousness
Shakiness
Lightheadedness
Hunger
Headache

Later Symptoms
Confusion
Disorientation
Lack of Coordination
Slurred Speech

Advanced Symptoms
Tremors
Convulsions
Loss of Consciousness

How to to Help Someone with Low Blood Sugar

For someone who is awake:

Offer one of the following:
1/2 cup juice
1/2 cup regular soda pop
(cannot be sugar-free)
5 Lifesavers or other
hard candy
1 cup milk
3 Glucose Tablets*
1/2 tube Insta-Glucose gel*
(*10 to 15 grams of carbohydrates)

Any of these should make
the person feel better in 10-15 min.
If not feeling better, repeat the
food or beverage

If no improvement in 15 min.,
take to a doctor or hospital or call 911

For Someone Who is Unconscious:

Give a glucagon shot
If no improvement in 15 min.,
take to a doctor or hospital
or call 911

If you can't give glucagon shot,
call 911

(SEE reproduction of glucagon insert, page 257-8)

INFORMATION FOR THE USER
Glucagon Emergency Kit
for Diabetic Insulin Reaction

BECOME FAMILIAR WITH THE FOLLOWING INSTRUCTIONS BEFORE AN EMERGENCY ARISES. DO NOT USE THIS KIT AFTER DATE STAMPED ON THE BOTTLE LABEL. IF YOU HAVE QUESTIONS CONCERNING THE USE OF THIS PRODUCT, CONSULT A DOCTOR.

GLUCAGON
FOR INJECTION, USP

IMPORTANT

- Act quickly. Prolonged unconsciousness may be harmful.
- Turn patient on his/her side to prevent patient from choking.
- The contents of the syringe are inactive. You must mix the contents of the syringe with the glucagon in the accompanying bottle before administering. (See DIRECTIONS FOR USE below.)
- Do not prepare Glucagon for Injection until you are ready to use it.

INDICATIONS FOR USE

Use glucagon to treat insulin coma or insulin reaction resulting from severe hypoglycemia (low blood sugar). Symptoms of severe hypoglycemia include disorientation, unconsciousness, and seizures or convulsions. Administer glucagon if (1) the patient is unconscious, (2) the patient is unable to eat sugar or a sugar-sweetened product, or (3) repeated administration of sugar or a sugar-sweetened product does not improve the patient's condition. Milder cases of hypoglycemia should be treated promptly by eating sugar or a sugar-sweetened product. (See INFORMATION ON HYPOGLYCEMIA below for more information on the symptoms of hypoglycemia.)

DIRECTIONS FOR USE
TO PREPARE GLUCAGON FOR INJECTION

1. Remove the flip-off seal from the bottle of glucagon. Wipe rubber stopper on bottle with alcohol swab.

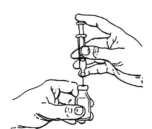

2. Remove the needle protector from the syringe, and inject the entire contents of the syringe into the bottle of glucagon.

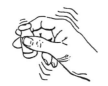

3. Remove syringe. Shake bottle gently until glucagon dissolves and the solution becomes clear. GLUCAGON SHOULD NOT BE USED UNLESS THE SOLUTION IS CLEAR AND OF A WATER-LIKE CONSISTENCY.

SEE NEXT SIDE FOR FURTHER DIRECTIONS

TO INJECT GLUCAGON
Use Same Technique as for Injecting Insulin

4. Using the same syringe, withdraw all of the solution (1-mg mark on syringe) from bottle. The plastic clip on the syringe will prevent the plunger from being pulled out of the syringe. The usual adult dose is 1 mg (1 unit). For children weighing less than 44 lb (20 kg), give 1/2 adult dose (0.5 mg). For children, withdraw 1/2 of the solution from the bottle (0.5-mg mark on syringe). **USING THE FOLLOWING DIRECTIONS, INJECT GLUCAGON IMMEDIATELY AFTER MIXING.**

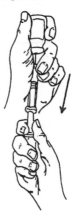

5. Cleanse injection site on buttock, arm, or thigh with alcohol swab.

6. Insert the needle into the loose tissue under the cleansed injection site, and inject all of the glucagon solution. THERE IS NO DANGER OF OVERDOSE. Apply light pressure at the injection site, and withdraw the needle. Press an alcohol swab against the injection site.

7. Turn the patient on his/her side. When an unconscious person awakens, he/she may vomit. Turning the patient on his/her side will prevent him/her from choking.

8. FEED THE PATIENT AS SOON AS HE/SHE AWAKENS AND IS ABLE TO SWALLOW. Give the patient a fast-acting source of sugar (such as a regular soft drink or orange juice) and a long-acting source of sugar (such as crackers and cheese or a meat sandwich). If the patient does not awaken within 15 minutes, give another dose of glucagon and INFORM A DOCTOR IMMEDIATELY.
   WARNING: THE PATIENT MAY BE IN A COMA FROM SEVERE HYPERGLYCEMIA (HIGH BLOOD GLUCOSE) RATHER THAN HYPOGLYCEMIA. IN SUCH A CASE, THE PATIENT WILL **NOT** RESPOND TO GLUCAGON AND REQUIRES IMMEDIATE MEDICAL ATTENTION.

9. Even if the glucagon revives the patient, his/her doctor should be promptly notified. A doctor should be notified whenever severe hypoglycemic reactions occur.

INFORMATION ON HYPOGLYCEMIA

Early symptoms of hypoglycemia (low blood glucose) include:

* sweating
* dizziness
* palpitation
* tremor
* hunger
* restlessness
* tingling in the hands, feet, lips, or tongue
* lightheadedness
* inability to concentrate
* headache
* drowsiness
* sleep disturbances
* anxiety
* blurred vision
* slurred speech
* depressive mood
* irritability
* abnormal behavior
* unsteady movement
* personality changes

If not treated, the patient may progress to severe hypoglycemia that can include:

* disorientation
* unconsciousness
* seizures
* death

The occurrence of early symptoms calls for prompt and, if necessary, repeated administration of some form of carbohydrate. Patients should always carry a quick source of sugar, such as candy mints or glucose tablets. The prompt treatment of mild hypoglycemic symptoms can prevent severe hypoglycemic reactions. If improvement does not occur or if administration of carbohydrate is impossible, glucagon should be given or the patient should be treated with the intravenous administration of glucose at a medical facility. Glucagon, a naturally occurring substance produced by the pancreas, is helpful because it enables the patient to produce his/her own blood glucose to correct the hypoglycemic state.

Literature revised August 3, 1995

ELI LILLY AND COMPANY • Indianapolis, IN 46285, USA
PA 0268 AMP   PRINTED IN USA

A SHORT Travel Appendix

Short (because every person with diabetes has different needs and has devised his or her own list of must-haves).

Still, it can't hurt to have a reminder of some of the stuff that has to be taken care of and toted. And, as a helpful family member or friend, you could offer to carry some of the extra gear, if you're able.

Travel by Air

Air travel has several special problems for anyone taking insulin (and to some extent) those who take blood-sugar-lowering pills:

1. Being at the mercy of the airline, its timetable, and food service schedule
2. Being unable to get to your luggage
3. Problems with customs re syringes and any medications
4. Traveling rapidly through many time zones

Traveling "Light"

These problems, and travel in general, mean you should revise your idea of what "traveling light" means. For the person with diabetes, lots of extras are essential. These could include:

- ❏ glucose tablets or gel
- ❏ non-perishable food sufficient *for an entire flight* or leg between train, bus, or auto stops
- ❏ card with important diabetes-related phrases (what to do in case of low blood sugar, etc.) in the language of the country or countries you are visiting
- ❏ a doctor's letter or prescription stating that insulin and needles are necessary
- ❏ doctor's phone and FAX numbers
- ❏ prescriptions for all medications
- ❏ medical insurance card and health insurance documents needed for reciprocal health agreements
- ❏ name of diabetes health care professional or diabetes center at destination
- ❏ name of English-speaking doctor if patient is traveling abroad (from International Association for Medical Assistance to Travellers: (716) 754-4883)
- ❏ blood glucose meter, strips, lancets, and log book
- ❏ at least two pairs of comfortable and broken-in shoes

- ❏ insulin (2-3 bottles of each type in different pieces of luggage. For example, one in his or her pockets, another in his or her carry-on, and one set in your carry-on)
- ❏ insulated container for insulin if likely to be in temperatures over 86° F or below freezing.
- ❏ disposable syringes with every insulin supply
- ❏ something to put sharps (used syringes and lancets) in until they can be disposed of appropriately
- ❏ diabetes pills   ❏ motion sickness pills or patches
- ❏ sunscreen   ❏ diarrhea medication
- ❏ first aid kit   ❏ ketone testing strips

Blood Sugar Level Scales Aren't Alike in Every Country

Your companion might need to communicate his blood sugar levels to a health care professional who isn't familiar with the measurements used in the country you're from. In the U.S., blood sugar is stated in milligrams per deciliter. In Canada, Europe, and most of the rest of the world milimols per liter is the norm.

To roughly convert from one system to the other, you can use this table:

mg/dl	30	60	90	120	150	180	210	270	300	330
mmo/L	1.7	3.3	5.0	6.7	8.3	10.0	11.7	15.0	16.7	18.3

For more exact conversions, use the formulas below:

To change milligrams per deciliter (usually abbreviated mg/dl) you:

multiply mg/dl by .05551 to get millimols/liter (mmol/L)

for example:
a blood glucose measurement of 120 would be 6.7 mmol/L
120 X .05551 = 6.6612 (rounded off, it's 6.7 mmol/L)

To change millimols/liter (mmol/L) into milligrams per deciliter (mg/dl) do this:

divide the level in mmol/L by .05551 to get mg/dl

for example:
a blood glucose measure of 4 mmol/L would be 72 mg/dl
4 mmol/L ÷ .05551 = 72 mg/dl

Prevention Trials For Type I Diabetes

The National Institutes of Health is looking for subjects for a prevention study. To be eligible to participate, you must:

1. Be between 3 and 45 years old and have a brother, sister, parent, son, or daughter who has Type I diabetes.

or

Be between the ages of 3 and 20 and have a niece, nephew, cousin, aunt, or uncle with Type I diabetes.

2. Have blood test results that show you are at high risk for developing Type I diabetes.

To get a list of the medical centers where testing is being done or to learn how a sample can by drawn by your physician, call the National Coordinating Center, in Miami:

(800)HALT-DM-1 or (800) 425-8361

Prevention Trials For Type II Diabetes

The National Institute of Diabetes and Digestive and Kidney Diseases is studying whether life-style changes or drugs can prevent or delay the onset of Type II diabetes in people who are at high risk. The trial will involve 4,000 people over age 25 who and have impaired glucose tolerance (blood sugar higher than normal but not high enough to qualify as diabetes).

You're a likely candidate (at high risk for developing diabetes) if any of these apply to you:

- Someone in you're family developed diabetes as an adult,
- You're overweight,
- You developed diabetes when you were pregnant,
- You've ever been told by your doctor that your blood sugar was a little bit high.

To request a brochure about the Diabetes Prevention Program or to learn where the 25 participating medical centers are located, call:

1(888)-DPP-JOIN or 1-(888)-377-5646

Auto Identification Bumper Sticker

A support group for people with diabetes produced this bumper sticker to alert police that a driver who may appear to be drunk could have low blood sugar and need medical help. It costs $2.50 by mail order. Orders of 25 or more are discounted.

DM Sticker Project
Albany's Hosp. Foundation for Community Health
1046 Sixth Avenue S.W.
Albany, OR 97321

World Wide Web

Lincoln Publishing Incorporated
Post Office Box 1499
Lake Oswego, OR 97035-0499

http://www.800books4u.com
(800) Books4u / (800) 266-5748
Tel: (503) 699-1000
Fax: (503) 699-2000

Lincoln's website has useful and interesting areas, including important pending health legislation; letters you can write to Congress and the President, along with information and references/links; details about media and in-person appearances by Janet Meirelles, and other authors of books we have available; other items you can order directly from the publisher; an order form; and "Letters to Lincoln."

American Diabetes Association
1660 Duke Street
Alexandria, VA 22314
Lots of information and periodicals.

http://www.diabetes.org
(800) 342-2383
(703) 549-1500

Juvenile Diabetes Foundation
120 Wall Street
New York, New York 10005

http://www.jdfcure.com
(800) 533-2873
Tel: (212) 785-9500
Fax: (212) 785-9595

Information, with an emphasis on type I diabetes research.

Newsletters

The Diabetes Is Not a Piece of Cake Newsletter - Janet Meirelles' monthly (almost) newsletter with food buying, current research, recipies, and much more. 11 issues a year ($12).

> Lincoln Publishing, Inc.   1-(800)-BOOKS-4-U
> P.O. Box 1499
> Lake Oswego, OR 97035-0499

The Challenge - Quarterly newsletter of the International Diabetic Athletes Association. Available to members ($15/yr):

> International Diabetic Athletes Assn.
> 1647–B West Bethany Home Rd.
> Phoenix, AZ 85015

Voice of the Diabetic is a publication of the National Federation of the Blind. This newsletter is of interest to those who are vision impaired and diabetic. It is free to any interested person. Also available on audio cassette for the blind.

> Voice of the Diabetic   (314)-875-8911
> 811 Cherry Street, Suite 309
> Columbia, MO 65201-4892

Magazines

Diabetes Forecast is the monthly magazine for members of the American Diabetes Association. Membership dues are $24 per year.

    American Diabetes Association, Inc.   1-(800)-232-3472
    1660 Duke Street
    Alexandria, Virginia 22314

Diabetes Interview is a monthly newspaper for the diabetes community. Subscriptions are $14 for 1 year, $24 for 2 years.

    Diabetes Interview   1-(800)-324-9434
    3715 Balboa Street
    San Francisco, CA 94121

Diabetes Self-Management is $18 per year for 6 issues. Canadian subscriptions are $30 per year in Canadian funds. Other countries are $36 per year in U.S. funds.

    Diabetes Self-Management
    R. A. Rapaport Publishing, Inc.   1-(800)-234-0923
    150 West 22nd Street
    New York, New York 10011

Two Types is a monthly diabetes magazine emphasizing lifestyle. U.S. subscriptions are $34.95 for 12 issues; Canada and Mexico, $50.95.

    Two Types   (800)-678-9691
    P.O. Box 1979
    Marion, OH 43306-2079

Cookbooks and Nutrition Guides

Meirelles, Janet, R.N., C.D.E., *Diabetes Is Not a Piece of Cake: THE COOKBOOK,* 167 pages, Lake Oswego, Lincoln Publishing, 1996.

    Over 100 pages of recipes for delicious, low fat, low sugar dishes. Everything from soup and appetizers to desserts that will delight without throwing blood sugar out of control.

    Starts with an introduction on healthy eating for folks with diabetes (and those without) including how to increase fiber, the scoop on portion sizes, do's and don't of feeding a guest with diabetes plus giving gifts of foods–with true caring.

Lund, JoAnna, *Healthy Exchanges Diabetic Cookbook,* JoAnna Lund lost 130 pounds with her creative recipes. All are low fat, low sugar, super-quick, and taste approved by her truck-driver husband. Delicious favorites made with convenience foods and easy-to-find ingredients. Every no-sweat healthy dish has diabetic exchanges plus a calorie, fat, and carbohydrate analysis by a registered dietitian.

Ulene, A., M.D. (Ed.), *The Nutribase Guide to Carbohydrates Calories & Fat In Your Food,* New York, Avery, 1995.

Ulene, A., M.D. (Ed.), *The Nutribase Nutrition Facts Desk Reference,* New York, Avery, 1995.

Warshaw, Hope S., *The Restaurant Companion: A Guide to Healthier Eating,* Surrey Books, 1995.

Miscellaneous Diabetes Books

American Diabetes Association. *Type II Diabetes: Your Healthy Living Guide.* Alexandria, VA. 1992.

Bailey, C. *The New Fit or Fat.* Boston: Houghton Mifflin, 1991.

Biermann, J., and Toohey, B. *The Diabetic's Book: All Your Questions Answered.* New York: Tarcher, 1994.

Biermann, J., and Toohey, B. *Diabetic's Total Health Book.* Los Angeles: Tarcher, 1992. (Also available in large print)

Biermann, J., and Toohey, B. *The Peripatetic Diabetic.* Boston: Houghton Mifflin, 1984.

Brackenridge, G.P. and Dolinar, R.O., MD, *Diabetes 101: Revised and Expanded 2nd Edition* (A Pure and Simple Guide for People Who Use Insulin, 1993.)

Brackenridge, G.P. and Rubin, R. *Sweet Kids: Diabetes Control and good nutrition with family peace,* 1996.

Curtis, J., *Living with Diabetes Complications.* Shippensburg, PA: Companion, 1993.

Edelwich, J. and Brodsky, A., *Diabetes: Caring For Your Emotions As Well As Your Health.* New York: Addison-Wesley, 1986.

Henry, L. and Johnson, K. *The Black Health Library Guide to Diabetes.* New York: Henry Holt, 1993.

Jovanovic, L., MD., Biermann, J., and Toohey, B. *The Diabetic Woman.* Los Angeles: Tarcher, 1996.

Lodewick, P., *A Diabetic Doctor Looks At Diabetes: His and Yours.* Massachusetts: R.M.I., 1993.

Lodewick, Peter, MD, Biermann, J., and Toohey, B., *The Diabetic Man.* 1996.

Milchovich, S., and Dunn-Long, B., *Diabetes Mellitus: A Practical Handbook.* Palo Alto: Bull Publishing, 1995.

Raymond, M., *The Human Side of Diabetes: Beyond Doctors, Diets, and Drugs*. Chicago: Noble, 1992.

Register, C., *Living With Chronic Illness*. New York: Bantam, 1989.

Rubin, R., PhD., Biermann, J., and Toohey, B. *Psyching Out Diabetes*. Los Angeles, Lowell House, 1992.

Tannenhaus, N., *What You Can Do About Diabetes*. New York: Dell, 1991.

Mail Order

Miscellaneous supplies: Meters and strips, pump supplies, insulin, creams, socks, artificial sweeteners in bulk, aids for visually impaired, traveling cases, sugar free cough meds, glucose tabs and gels, impotence treatments, armchair exercise video, books, and more.

Diabetes Supply Club	in Portland	(503) 287-9303
3510 N.E. 57th Street	outside Portland, Oregon 1-800-358-2525	
Portland, OR 97213		

Booklets, books, and video tape can be borrowed or bought from the American Diabetes Association. Find your local affiliate by looking in the white pages under "diabetes."

Lincoln Publishing Incorporated (the publisher of this book) offers books, newsletters, and other items that Ms. Meirelles recommends. Call, write, or e-mail for a complete catalog and order form– or take a look at the LPI webpage.

Lincoln Publishing, Inc.   http://www.800books4u.com
  Post Office Box 1499   (800) Books4u / (800) 266-5748
  Lake Oswego, OR 97035-0499   Tel: (503) 699-1000
                                      Fax: (503) 699-2000

Living With Diabetes Complications ($15.95, postage is included) can be ordered from Lincoln Publishing or from:

Outreach Enterprises	(503) 224-9857
2221 S.W. 1st Ave., Suite 2322	
Portland, OR 97201-5009	

Prana publications handles all the Biermann and Toohey books and many more of the newest and the best. For a free newsletter with the latest on diabetes plus book ordering information call or write:

Prana Publications	1-800-735-7726
5623 Matilija Ave.	Fax: (818) 786-7359
Van Nuys, CA 91401	E-Mail: prana2@aol.com

Booklets and books on diabetes and other health topics are available from Chronimed Publishing.

Chronimed Publishing 1-800-848-2793, ext 861
P.O. Box 47945
Minneapolis, Minnesota 55447-9727

Medical Jewelry

Bracelet or neck chain emblem engraved with health information and 24-hour hot line number with medical facts, physician, and contact information. The charge is $35.00 and up for lifetime emergency hot line service, custom engraved emblem, and wallet card.

Medic Alert Foundation 1 (800)-432-5378
2323 Colorado Ave.
Turlock, CA 95380

Special Cruises for Diabetics

All the fun of a cruise with informative workshops on diabetes conducted by the Joslin Diabetes Center. For information of coming cruise destinations contact:

Specialty Group Cruises 1 (800)-228-0558
400 Washington St.
Braintree, MA 02184

Informational Kits for Schools

Managing Diabetes: A Guide For Schools #35-MDGS-O
The Oregon Affiliate of the ADA developed this publication to provide support and assistance to school personnel to assure that students with diabetes have a positive and safe school experience. Written in a concise and clear manner, this guide provides action plans for parents and individual school personnel (e.g. principal, teacher, health personnel, coaches, and food service personnel). Also included are age specific charts describing low and high blood sugar reactions (suitable for laminating and posting) emergency procedures, and recipes for special occasions. $4.00 (postage and handling are included)

American Diabetes Association Tel: (503) 736-2700
Oregon Affiliate, Inc. Fax: (503) 736-2774
380 S.E. Spokane St., Suite 110
Portland, OR 97202

For the Resources You've Discovered –

_____

_____

_____

_____

_____

_____

_____

_____

_____

_____

_____

_____

_____

_____

_____

To order additional copies of *the cookbook* ($12.95 each) or copies of *Diabetes is not a piece of cake* ($15.95 each) you may call our order number with your VISA or MASTERCARD or the information requested below with your payment.

(800) BOOKS-4-U
[(800) 266-5748].

Shipping and handling for first book is $3.00, each additional is $0.75. Second day air delivery is available for only $3.50 extra. Payable in U.S. funds. No cash orders accepted. Prices, shipping & handling may change without notice. At time of printing no sales tax is due. Call about quantity purchases.

Photocopy this coupon

LINCOLN PUBLISHING INCORPORATED

http://www.800books4u.com	Orders: (800) BOOKS-4-U
Post Office Box 1499	Tel: (503) 699-1000
Lake Oswego, OR 97035-1499 USA	Fax: (503) 699-2000

Book(s) ordered _____

Name_____   Book total $_____

Address _____   shpg & hndlg $_____

City _____   Next day air $_____

State/Zip _____   Total amt due $_____

Bill my: ❏ VISA ❏ MASTERCARD expires _____

card # _____

Signature _____
or enclosed is my: ❏ check ❏ money order

Subscription to Ms. Meirelles' monthly diabetes newsletter is also available. Lincoln Publishing also makes available other books and items, some of which are difficult to obtain from other sources. Please contact us for a catalog and for international orders.

Letters to the author should be addressed in care of the publisher, and if a reply is requested, included a self-addressed postage paid (#9 or #10) business envelope.

The author is available for speaking engagements.

Glossary

acesulfame-K - artificial, noncaloric sweetener sold as Sweet One and Sunette. Does not lose its sweetness in baking.

acidosis - harmful build-up of acids in the blood which can be caused by burning of fats when there is insufficient insulin to "process" sugar needed for energy.

adrenaline (also called epinephrine) - hormone produced by the adrenal gland which signals the liver to release stored glucose.

aerobic exercise - exercise in which the heart and lungs are able to supply enough oxygen for the effective use of stored energy. This level is usually reached when the heart is beating at 65-80% of its maximum rate.

alpha cells - cells in the pancreas which produce glucagon, a hormone which acts to raise blood glucose.

anaerobic exercise - exercise in which there is insufficient oxygen supplied for the effective use of stored energy. Exercise at this level can be only done for short periods.

apple-shaped body type - body type with most excess fat above the waist. People with this upper body fat are at higher risk of heart disease and stoke.

arteriosclerosis - narrowing and hardening of artery walls which reduces the arteries' ability to carry sufficient oxygen-rich blood to the cells. Narrowing is caused by the formation of raised areas in the inner lining of the arteries. These deposits are especially common in people with high concentrations of cholesterol in their blood.

aspartame - artificial noncaloric sweetener sold as Equal or Nutrasweet. Cannot be used for baking as it loses it sweetness at high temperatures for prolonged time.

autoimmune disorder - malfunction of the body's defense against invading organisms which makes antibodies that harm the body's own cells.

basal rate - constant, low insulin output from the pancreas or an insulin pump to provide between-meal insulin needs.

beta cells - cells in the islets of Langerhans of the pancreas which produce insulin.

blood sugar meter or monitor - device that measures the amount of sugar in a drop of blood placed on a specially-treated strip.

bolus - extra insulin from the pancreas or an insulin pump before meals or snacks.

calorie - measure of energy or heat. Energy content of foods and energy used to perform activities is measured in kilocalories (thousands of calories) but is usually shortened to "calories".

carbohydrate - one of the three classes of energy-producing nutrients (fat and protein are the other two). In the intestine, carbohydrate is changed into a simple sugar then absorbed into the bloodstream and is used by cells for immediate energy or stored for future use. Has 4 calories per gram.

cardiovascular conditioning - progressive strengthening of the heart, lungs, and circulatory system by aerobic exercise.

cardiovascular disease - disease of the heart, blood vessels and blood circulation. Includes heart attacks, stroke, high blood pressure, and blockages.

cataract - loss of transparency of the lens of the eye.

certified diabetes educator - nurse, dietitian, social worker, physician, pharmacist, or exercise physiologist who has done direct diabetes education for at least 2000 hours and has passed a national exam of competency in diabetes and teaching. Retaking of the exam is required every 5 years to maintain the certificate.

cesarean delivery - surgical operation to deliver a baby through an incision in the abdomen.

cholesterol - blood fat produced by the liver from saturated fats or absorbed from foods like eggs and dairy products which are rich in cholesterol. High levels can lead to increased risk of heart disease and stroke.

control solution - liquid with a pre-determined sugar level that is used in place of a drop of blood to test the accuracy of a blood glucose meter.

cyclamate - artificial sweetener not approved by FDA for sale in the U.S.

dehydration - serious condition in which the body's water content falls to a low level. Especially likely to occur during illness when water may be lost through diarrhea, vomiting, or increased urination due to high blood sugar.

diabetes insipidus - is a rare deficiency of a pituitary antidiuretic hormone (ADH) or lack of response by the kidneys to the hormone. Without ADH, the kidneys make too much urine, causing extreme thirst. Diabetes insipidus is not related to and has nothing besides the symptoms of thirst and frequent urination in common with diabetes mellitus.

diabetes mellitus - disorder of metabolism which produces high blood sugar levels. It results from insufficient insulin production or poor utilization of insulin.

diabetic food - food that is low in sugar but may have other carbohydrates and fat. Cannot be eaten in unlimited quantities.

dialysis - process of filtering blood to remove toxic materials and maintain fluid and chemical balance as a substitute for failed or partially functioning kidneys.

dietetic food - food that is higher or lower in some element (salt, etc.) but is not necessarily low in sugar or designed for people with diabetes.

dietitian - person trained in nutrition. A registered dietitian (R.D.) has passed an exam which tests competency and is licensed by the state in which he or she practices.

digestive enzymes - proteins, produced primarily by the pancreas, and secreted into the small intestine, that break foods down into chemicals that can be absorbed and used.

endocrine gland - gland which produces hormones that are released into the blood and which have effects on distant parts of the body. The pancreas is an endocrine gland.

endocrinologist - physician who specializes in disorders of the endocrine glands. Most endocrinologists treat diabetes more than any other glandular problem.

end-stage kidney disease - advanced kidney disease requiring the use of artificial blood filtering (see dialysis). Symptoms may include nausea, vomiting, weakness, and loss of appetite.

enzymes - specific proteins produced by cells to cause or speed up chemical reactions.

exchange system - division of foods into groups that are nearly equal in calories, carbohydrate, protein, and fat. Foods in one group can be exchanged for any food *within the same group*.

exercise physiologist - professional trained in exercise science or exercise physiology who is able to design an exercise program, based on treadmill work or other tests, that specifies frequency, duration, intensity, and type of exercise. Also evaluates responses of blood sugar to exercise and assists in education of patients.

fasting blood sugar - sugar concentration in the blood when no food has been eaten for 8 hours or more. A normal value from a sample from a vein and sent to a lab is 70-115, a normal finger-stick value on a blood glucose meter is 60-100.

fat - one of the three classes of energy-producing food (carbohydrates and proteins are the other two). Has 9 calories per gram.

fiber - indigestible parts of plants. May help lower cholesterol, blood sugar, and promote better intestinal function.

fructose - a sugar found in fruit that causes less rise in blood sugar when used instead of table sugar to sweeten foods. Has been found along with table sugar to increase levels of triglycerides.

gangrene - death of tissue caused by insufficient blood supply.

gestational diabetes - diabetes that occurs during pregnancy (usually after the 24th week). It is caused by hormonal changes that cause the body to require more insulin than can be naturally produced. Diet, and sometimes insulin, are necessary usually only until the birth. Treatment is necessary to prevent the birth of a dangerously large baby or a premature birth.

glaucoma - eye disorder in which increased pressure inside the eye can damage the optic nerve, resulting in blindness. Early diagnosis and treatment are essential.

glucagon - hormone produced by the alpha cells in the pancreas. When blood sugar levels get low, it stimulates the breakdown of glycogen (a carbohydrate stored in the liver and muscles) into sugar. An injectable form is available by prescription for correcting low blood sugar of someone who is unconscious.

glucose - form of sugar most used by cells for energy. Ninety percent of carbohydrates are changed into glucose.

glucose gel - glucose preparation in a gel form. Comes in tubes that hold 30 grams glucose. The contents are squeezed into the mouth to correct a low blood sugar.

Glucose Tablet - tablet that contains 5 grams of glucose. Two or three are chewed when blood sugar is low.

glycemic index - list of different foods' effect on blood sugar compared with glucose or white bread.

glycogen - form of carbohydrate stored in the liver and muscles. It can be converted back into glucose when needed.

glycohemoglobin - portions of a red blood cell's hemoglobin that collect sugar molecules. Measurement of glycohemoglobin indicates how often the blood sugar level was high.

glycosylated hemoglobin test - test which measures blood sugar levels over last two months. (See glycohemoglobin, above)

gram - unit of weight of the metric system. A penny weighs 3 grams.

HDL - "good" type of cholesterol. Initials stand for high density lipoprotein. A higher proportion of HDL seems to protect against cardiovascular disease.

hemoglobin A1C - portion of the hemoglobin of the red blood cell that collects sugar molecules. Same as glycosylated hemoglobin.

high blood sugar (hyperglycemia) - higher than normal amount of sugar in the blood. Two hours or more after a meal, blood sugar should be, at most 180, but ideally less than 140.

honeymoon phase - period when a person with newly diagnosed Type I diabetes may need little or no injected insulin because their own insulin-producing cells have temporarily resumed production. Occasionally this period lasts as long as a year but it usually lasts only a few weeks.

hormone - chemical produced by a gland which is released into the blood stream. It can affect a part far from the gland that produced it. Insulin is a hormone.

hydrogenated - oil or fat that has had hydrogen atoms added to it

through a chemical process to make it more solid. Solidifying a polyunsaturated oil causes it to lose much of the health benefit of being polyunsaturated.

hyperbaric chamber - compartment which contains a higher than normal atmospheric pressure. This allows more oxygen to be carried by the blood and can be useful in the treatment of gangrene. Also used to treat divers for the bends.

hyperglycemia - higher than normal amount of sugar in the blood (over 180, 2 hours or more after a meal is high blood sugar. Some physicians would prefer it be under 140).

hypersomotic coma - a coma caused by very high blood sugar resulting in dehydration. May occur in someone with Type II diabetes under the same conditions that would cause ketoacidosis in someone with Type I diabetes.

hypertension (high blood pressure) - higher than normal blood pressure within the arteries. A reading greater than 140/90 is usually considered high blood pressure.

hypoglycemia - lower than normal amount of sugar in the blood. Below 60 would be considered low.

impotence - inability to achieve or maintain an erection.

insoluble fiber - part of plant (such as wheat bran) that does not dissolve in water and is not digested. Helps digestion.

insulin - hormone produced by the pancreas. It is essential for the maintenance of the proper blood sugar level and for the metabolism of food, especially carbohydrates.

insulin-dependent diabetes (IDDM) - (Also called Type I or juvenile-onset diabetes). Diabetes which usually occurs before the age of 20. Is brought on by the complete destruction of the insulin-producing cells in the pancreas. Treatment requires insulin replacement by injection.

insulin pump - beeper-sized battery-powered device which delivers insulin through a tube into a needle left under the skin in one place for 2-3 days at a time. A computer programmed by the wearer regulates small continuous basal amounts between meals and larger bolus amounts at meals and snacks.

insulin receptor - chemical "locks" on cells that react to insulin, allowing sugar to enter the cell. A deficiency in the number of receptors is a cause of sugar accumulating in the blood in Type II diabetes.

insulin resistance - ineffective use of insulin that occurs in Type II diabetes. May be caused by too few receptors (see insulin receptor, above) or poor function of receptors or some unknown disfunction within the cell.

intravenous (I.V.) fluids - sterile fluids given through a needle or catheter into a vein.

islets of Langerhans - clusters of cells in the pancreas that contain alpha cells (produce glucagon) and beta cells (produce insulin) that regulate blood sugar.

ketoacidosis - abnormal acid condition caused by the accumulation of ketones which are produced when there is insufficient insulin present in the body for glucose to be used for energy. The use of fats as an emergency energy source, produces toxic ketones. This can result in dehydration and chemical and fluid imbalances which can be fatal if not treated.

ketones - by-products of the use of fat as an energy source when insulin is not available. (See ketoacidosis, above)

ketonuria - presence of ketones in urine. Moderate to large amounts may indicate ketoacidosis.

kidneys - organs which filter the blood, regulate fluid and salt balance, remove toxins and produce urine.

lactose - sugar found naturally in milk.

lancets - small, pointed, "needles" used to puncture the skin to get a drop of blood for a blood sugar test. They are usually held in a pen-sized holder which quickly releases the lancet at the touch of a button, controlling the depth of the puncture.

laser - device that produces a concentrated beam of light. It is used in the treatment of diabetic retinopathy to prevent bleeding from weak blood vessels. It is also used to re-attach the retina if torn.

lipids - word meaning *fats*. Commonly used when speaking of cholesterol and triglycerides which are frequently overabundant in the blood. High levels of lipids have been found to be present more often in people who have had heart attacks and strokes.

liver - organ which manufactures and regulates levels of many of the body's chemicals. One of its functions is the storage of glucose when it is not needed, and its reformation from glycogen and protein.

LDL - Low density lipoprotein, also called "bad" cholesterol. When LDL cholesterol is present in the blood in large amounts, the risk of developing heart disease and strokes increases.

low blood sugar (hypoglycemia) - lower than normal amount of sugar in the blood. Below 60 is usually considered low.

meal plan - personalized eating plan which includes quantity, types of foods, and timing. Age, weight, medication, and other factors influence these three components.

medical identification - bracelet, anklet, or necklace which identifies the wearer as a diabetic. Some describe treatment or give a toll-free phone number which can be called for medical information.

metabolism - sum of all the chemical changes that take place in the body. Metabolism of food refers to how food is broken down into smaller parts as when some of a potato becomes sugar in the blood. It also refers to the opposite process - taking smaller chemical units like sugar and making them into larger units such as fat tissue.

metformin - diabetes pill that reduces insulin resistance and improves cholesterol and triglyceride levels.

microalbumin - urine test for any tiny amount of protein. It's presence may signal early kidney disease.

milligram - one-thousandth of a gram. A penny weighs 3000 milligrams or 3 grams.

monounsaturated oil - oil that seems to be less harmful than solid (saturated) fats. Monounsaturated oils include olive oil and canola oil.

neonatologist - physician who specializes in the care of newborn babies.

nephropathy - kidney disease. (See end-stage kidney disease).

neuropathy - disease of the nerves. Symptoms in arms and legs include numbness, tingling, coldness, and pain. Almost any part of the body can be affected by this complication of diabetes.

normal blood sugar - Usually considered to be about 80-120 mg/dl (milligrams per deciliter).

NPH insulin - intermediate-acting insulin which starts working in 1-2 hours, has a peak of action between 6-12 hours, and lasts from 18-26 hours. The letters stand for Neutral Protamine Hagedorn. Neutral, because it is neither chemically an acid nor a base, protamine (now isophane), which is added to extend the time it takes to be absorbed, and Hagedorn, the name of the inventor.

noninsulin-dependent diabetes (NIDDM) - also Type II diabetes or adult-onset diabetes. This type usually occurs after age 40. Eighty to ninety-five percent of people with diabetes have this form. Treatment includes diet, exercise, and may require oral medication. Insulin is needed by about 30% of NIDDM patients.

obesity - condition of having too much body fat. Usually a person must be at least 20% over maximum desirable weight to be considered obese. Obesity is present in about 80% of people who get Type II diabetes.

ophthalmologist - physician who specializes in treating diseases of the eyes.

optometrist - health care provider trained to measure vision and fit eye glasses and contact lenses. Most states do not allow optometrists to use medication to dilate pupils so they are unable to perform the thorough eye exam necessary to detect diabetic eye complications.

oral diabetes pills (sulfonylureas and metformin) - medication which may improve blood sugar levels. Not oral insulin. (See insulin receptor and insulin resistance).

pancreas - abdominal organ which produces the hormone insulin. It also makes the hormone glucagon which raises blood sugar and digestive enzymes which help digestion.

pancreatitis - inflammation of the pancreas which may result in damage to the pancreas. Occasionally, some or all the gland must be surgically removed resulting in a shortage or complete lack of insulin, glucagon, and pancreatic digestive enzymes.

pear-shaped body type - body type with excess fat below the waist resulting in a pear-shape. Fat in the thighs and buttocks is less likely to result in heart disease and strokes than fat above the waist. (See appleshaped body type).

pediatrician - physician that specializes in the physical development and medical care of children.

plaque - fatty deposit on the inside of artery walls which results in a narrowing which can lead to an inadequate blood supply in the area the artery supplies. Plaque is formed from LDL cholesterol and other materials. Eventually plaque can thicken until it blocks the vessel or a piece can break off, causing blockage somewhere else.

podiatrist - a doctor (although not an MD) who specializes in the prevention and treatment of foot disorders including foot ulcers and infections of people with diabetes. Is qualified to perform surgery on foot conditions.

polyunsaturated oil - an oil that lacks two or more hydrogen atoms. Thought to be less likely to cause clogged arteries than solid (saturated) fats. Polyunsaturated oils include corn and safflower oils.

postprandial - following a meal. Postprandial blood sugar testing is sometimes recommended to learn how a particular meal affected blood sugar.

preeclampsia - serious condition of pregnancy characterized by increased blood pressure, headaches, fluid retention, nausea and vomiting, abdominal pain, visual disturbances, and protein in the urine. Preeclampsia is more frequent in women with diabetes. It may lead to the more serious condition, eclampsia, which can cause seizures and may require emergency delivery to save the mother and fetus.

proliferative retinopathy - serious diabetic complication of the retina of the eyes. Laser treatment is frequently successful in preventing its progression to blindness.

protein - one of the three food types that can provide energy (the other two are carbohydrate and fat). Protein is primarily used to build tissue. Excess protein is turned into fat. Protein has 4 calories per gram.

pump - beeper-sized battery-powered device which delivers insulin through a tube into a needle left under the skin in one place for 2-3 days at a time. A computer inside the pump, programmed by the wearer, regulates small continuous basal amounts between meals and larger bolus amounts at meals and snacks.

retina - the light-sensitive tissue lining the interior of the eye. It contains special nerve cells which convert light energy into nerve impulses. (See proliferative retinopathy)

retinopathy - any disease of the retina. Background retinopathy does not usually impair vision but shows that diabetic changes are occurring. More serious are preproliferative and proliferative retinopathy. See proliferative retinopathy.

saccharin - an artificial sweetener that has no calories. May be used for cooking and baking.

saturated fat - fats which are solid at room temperature. These tend to contribute more to plaque formation in arteries which may lead to cardiovascular disease.

simple carbohydrate - sugar.

soluble fiber - part of plant foods (beans, oats, etc.) that dissolves in water in the intestine. Improves digestion, blood cholesterol level, and slows absorption of sugar from the intestine.

subcutaneous tissue - fatty layer below the skin into which insulin is injected.

sucrose - table sugar, beet sugar, cane sugar. Is used to make granulated, powdered, and brown sugars.

sugar - simple form of carbohydrate. When dozens of sugar units are joined together a complex carbohydrate or starch is formed.

sugar-free - term used by food processors which may mean it does not contain sucrose (white table sugar) but may contain any of several other forms of sugar. Does *not* mean it is carbohydrate-free or glucose-free.

sulfonylureas - diabetes pills which lower blood sugar. These are not an oral form of insulin. They may stimulate insulin production, decrease liver release of sugar, and facilitate insulin action on the cell which allows glucose to enter the cell more easily. (See insulin receptor and insulin resistance).

syringe - temporary container of liquid medication to which a hollow needle is attached. By inserting the needle into the body and then pushing on the piston portion of the syringe, the liquid is forced through the needle and into the body.

target range - an effective exercise exertion level. The range is 65%-80% of maximum heart rate (220 minus age).

Type I diabetes (insulin-dependent, IDDM, or juvenile-onset diabetes) type of diabetes which usually occurs before the age of 20. Is brought on by the complete destruction of the insulin-producing cells in the pancreas. Treatment requires insulin replacement by injection.

Type II diabetes (non-insulin dependent diabetes, NIDDM, or adult-onset diabetes) type of diabetes which usually occurs after age 40. Eighty to ninety percent of people with diabetes have this form. Treatment includes diet, exercise, and may require oral medication. Insulin is needed for about 30% of NIDDM cases.

ultralente insulin - long-acting insulin which begins acting in 4-6 hours, has it's peak action between 18-25 hours, and lasts up to 36 hours.

units - how insulin is prescribed and measured. One cubic centimeter (cc) of insulin has 100 units.

unsaturated fat - oil that is not saturated (full) of hydrogen atoms. Considered to be less harmful than saturated fat.

Index

Here's Our Contact Information:

For catalog and/or ordering information, please also see page 268, or visit our world wide website:

http://www.800books4u.com
e-mail: info@800books4u.com
Lincoln Publishing Incorporated
Tel: (503) 699-1000 / Fax: (503) 699-2000
catalog requests & retail orders: (800) Books4u [800-266-5748]
Post Office Box 1499
Lake Oswego, OR 97035-0499